MAY - 3 2019

3 1994 01582 6370

SANTA ANA PUBLIC LIBRARY

P9-CJC-402

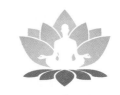

Essential Oils
for
Mindfulness
and
Meditation

"There is a unique way to enhance psychological well-being waiting to be explored. This book tells you how meditation and aromatherapy, classic tools for modifying the mind, can work together to maintain a state of calm and insight. Familiar oils like rose and frankincense add serenity and inspiration to the practice of mindfulness meditation. Diffusing an essential oil during meditation practice can even return your awareness to that meditative mode if you smell the aromatic oil again later.

The author is an aromatherapist who not only uses essential oils professionally but also conducts research into the effects of these powerful plant ingredients. The reader will find out how knowledge of traditional practice and subjective experience, backed by scientific evidence, is an ideal path for discovery; how mindfulness meditation and essential oil inhalation relieve anxiety or calm the mind, as explained from the perspectives of ancient history, religious practices, and modern complementary medical practice. Scientific studies involving human subjects and essential oils tested in laboratory models are described in easy-to-digest detail that adds value and validity.

Advice on how to use the pure essential oils comes with a thorough briefing on dose and safety—a prerequisite for these concentrated and potent plant extracts. In passing, learning about the many everyday food, drink, and cosmetic products that contain essential oils is an eye-opener on the hidden influences on the mind and body.

This book is bound to have a long-lasting impact on both meditation and aromatherapy practices, thanks to its inspired author, Heather Dawn Godfrey."

ELAINE PERRY, PH.D., PROFESSOR EMERITUS OF
NEUROSCIENCE AT NEWCASTLE UNIVERSITY

"*Essential Oils for Mindfulness and Meditation* fills an important gap in the field of essential oils. Where many other books are contented with the properties and the handling of oils, Heather Godfrey provides us with a profound scientific background of the different oils and opens up the field toward awareness and meditation. This book is a wonderful guide to using essential oils as valuable helpers for everyday life, as a source of knowledge for well-being professionals, and for a deeper understanding of oneself and nature."

EWALD KLIEGEL, AUTHOR OF
CRYSTAL WANDS AND *HOLISTIC REFLEXOLOGY*

"This interesting book melds the science and alchemy of essential oils and their use in meditation with a mix of personal anecdotes and evidence. Taking the reader on a journey through these highly topical disciplines, it is a timely reminder and how-to guide of the importance of stepping back from the maelstrom of modern life to find a sensible inner balance."

SOPHIE [PETIT-ZEMAN] OLSZOWSKI, PH.D., AUTHOR OF
DOCTOR, WHAT'S WRONG? MAKING THE NHS HUMAN AGAIN
AND EDITOR, NHS RESEARCHER, AND DIRECTOR OF
SPZ ASSOCIATES LTD.

Essential Oils

for

Mindfulness

and

Meditation

Relax, Replenish, and Rejuvenate

615.3219 GOD
Godfrey, Heather Dawn
Essential oils for
  mindfulness and
  meditation

                                $16.99
CENTRAL   31994015826370

Heather Dawn Godfrey, PGCE, BSc

Healing Arts Press
Rochester, Vermont

Healing Arts Press
One Park Street
Rochester, Vermont 05767
www.HealingArtsPress.com

Healing Arts Press is a division of Inner Traditions International

Copyright © 2018 by Heather Dawn Godfrey

All rights reserved. No part of this book may be reproduced or utilized in any form or by any means, electronic or mechanical, including photocopying, recording, or by any information storage and retrieval system, without permission in writing from the publisher.

Note to the reader: This book is intended as an informational guide. The remedies, approaches, and techniques described herein are meant to supplement, and not to be a substitute for, professional medical care or treatment. They should not be used to treat a serious ailment without prior consultation with a qualified health care professional.

Library of Congress Cataloging-in-Publication Data
Names: Godfrey, Heather Dawn, author.
Title: Essential oils for mindfulness and meditation : relax, replenish, and rejuvenate / Heather Dawn Godfrey, PGCE, BSc.
Description: Rochester, Vermont : Healing Arts Press, [2018] | Includes bibliographical references and index.
Identifiers: LCCN 2018012261 (print) | LCCN 2018012914 (ebook) | ISBN 9781620557624 (paperback) | ISBN 9781620557631 (ebook)
Subjects: LCSH: Aromatherapy. | Essences and essential oils—Therapeutic use. | Mind and body. | Meditation. | BISAC: HEALTH & FITNESS / Aromatherapy. | BODY, MIND & SPIRIT / Meditation. | SELF-HELP / Spiritual.
Classification: LCC RM666.A68 G63 2018 (print) | LCC RM666.A68 (ebook) | DDC 615.3/219—dc23
LC record available at https://lccn.loc.gov/2018012261

Printed and bound in the United States by Versa Press, Inc.

10 9 8 7 6 5 4 3 2 1

Text design and layout by Virginia Scott Bowman
This book was typeset in Garamond Premier Pro and Gill Sans with Coats and Frutiger used as display typefaces
Diagrams on pages 37, 47, 48, 50, and 105 by W. Dowell and D. Smith, www.coastlinecreative.co.uk, 2017

To send correspondence to the author of this book, mail a first-class letter to the author c/o Inner Traditions • Bear & Company, One Park Street, Rochester, VT 05767, and we will forward the communication, or contact the author directly at **www.aromantique.co.uk.**

Contents

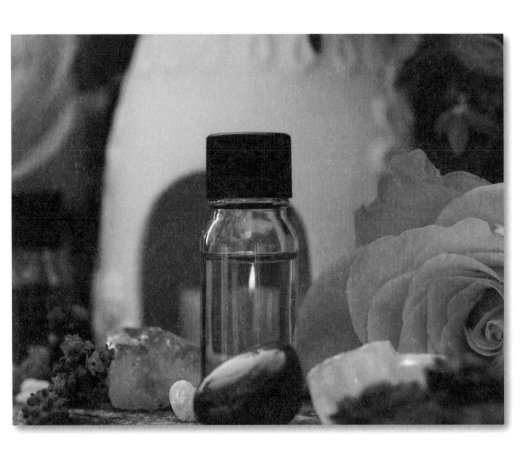

Preface

I was introduced to essential oils many years ago, when I worked for Robert Tisserand in London, during those early days when he first began developing his business, the Aromatic Oil Company, later Tisserand Aromatherapy. Then, I was a teenager, naive and idealistic, believing that I had so many years ahead, my life spreading out before me with endless possibility. So, when a friend beckoned me to join her in Corsica to work for a season, I went without hesitation, assuming I could simply pick up the threads when I was ready to return. Within a year, however, I was married and expecting my first child, my path decided and etched to a distant horizon.

One day, four beautiful children and some years later, I serendipitously found myself in a bookshop, waiting for a friend. Browsing the shelves in front of me, I noticed with pleasant surprise a book written by Robert, *The Art of Aromatherapy*. Intrigued, I flicked through the pages. Memories instantly flooded through me; the air I breathed seemed suddenly imbued with the scent of rose, ylang ylang, and chamomile. I recalled, as if only the day before, weighing dried chamomile and rose flowers and packing small brown bottles of essential oils with Robert and Jonathon ("Jack" and "Hans," as they were known then). I remembered the indulgent ambience the scents created—sweet, spicy, earthy, leafy, fruity, woody, floral, deeply rich, or playfully light—permeating every corner of the space, dispelling the dank background smell in the small old building we occupied then.

From that chance moment in the bookshop, revisiting the comfort, the familiarity, the tingle of excitement I felt, my inspiration was rekindled. My children were growing, and it was time to pick up the threads I had started to weave and complete the journey I had begun during those early years in London.

I earned a joint honors degree in counseling and complementary medicine at the University of Salford and master's certificates in integrated mindfulness and supervision of counseling and therapeutic relationships, going on to work in several capacities at the College of Health and Social Care at the University of Salford, including running the aromatherapy clinic for staff and students. I've also offered essential oil therapy in private practice for over 25 years.

I have had the good fortune to work with a range of clients (parents, grandparents, caregivers, teachers, researchers, managers, nurses, acupuncturists, counselors, and a variety of health-care professionals, among others) who have sought treatments for many different reasons. These include balancing physical and psycho-emotional well-being while working in demanding roles; managing stress or a stress-related condition, such as insomnia, mild depression, or anxiety; and support during challenging life events such as bereavement, job loss, or relationship breakdown, and, conversely, exciting events such as moving, changing jobs, or getting married. Sometimes it is for the simple but possibly most significant reason of all: to relax and enhance a sense of well-being.

Indeed, the inspiration to write this book evolved from observing my clients' responses to the scent of essential oils. I observed how the experience of aroma absorption and perception drew their attention and awareness into the moment. I also noticed how those moments were enriched as the scent permeated their psychic being and appeared to trigger a psycho-emotional response and effect. These responses were initially observed through a softening of facial expression and calmer breathing, after which clients reported their experience of increased energy, clearer thinking, and a sense of feeling relaxed and grounded. Their experiences have also been substantiated by measurable physiological responses in the nervous system.

Just as my connection to essential oils began many years ago, so did my relationship with meditation. When I learned to meditate, meditation was regarded as a fringe or hippie-type practice, encapsulated and epitomized by media images of the Beatles sitting with Maharishi Mahesh Yogi, developer of Transcendental Meditation. Meditation has not changed my destiny or my life's lessons, but it is an invaluable tool, consistently grounding my sense of reality, anchoring my psyche when I feel insecure, calming my racing mind, and uncluttering my perspective. I do not meditate every day, but whenever I do, the experience is unconditional, unfailing, always "just there," if I choose to notice, to focus my awareness.

Mindfulness is a meditative construct similarly applied as a tool, to the same end. It is an ancient practice, steeped in Buddhist philosophy, which nonetheless currently occupies the foreground of vogue acceptance as a nonreligious, cost-effective, destressing, antianxiety, antidepressant tool. It is increasingly embraced by mainstream health care as a viable self-help remedy that may be safely applied independently or alongside conventional treatments.

At my age, I am aware that there is no magic formula, and that life is a journey. We each travel on our own path, which may sometimes be easy and sometimes difficult to tread. However, there are positive and negative ways of coping with the stresses and joys of everyday life. Around the world and through the ages, meditation and mindfulness have been practiced and valued as among the most positive and effective methods.

Companions of the meditative process and remedies in their own right, essential oils play an invaluable complementary role, particularly when we utilize their psycho-emotional properties such as their ability to uplift, brace, and ground. These qualities, among many other significant ones, are simple yet important when dealing with everyday life. Through my clinical practice, observing my clients' responses to essential oils, and my own experience, I notice how enriching this relationship is, how practical and pleasurable, healing and uplifting, and how this in turn may also translate into a healthy sense of well-being. Essential oils appear to be a multidynamic gift presented by nature—offered, it seems, to accompany our journey through life, through the ups and downs and the joys and challenges, like a supportive friend.

Acknowledgments

My sincere thanks and gratitude are extended to my daughter April Sandrene Tatlock, my godmother May Copp, my brother Stephen Godfrey, Jane Logie, Linda Manzioni, Sonraya Grace, Laura Joyce, and Ian Prudence, for their unconditional support, belief, and encouragement.

Photographs featured in this book were taken with kind permission at Compton Acres Gardens (Poole, Dorset, UK BH13 7ES, www.comptonacres.co.uk); my thanks and appreciation are extended to Joseph Coogan, gardener, for sharing his wealth of knowledge and expertise, and Bernard Merna, owner of the gardens, for allowing me access, often before the gardens were open in the morning, to take photographs to illustrate my books. Examples of essential oil–bearing plants (along with many other herbaceous and medicinal plants) located within the gardens include angelica (*Angelica officinalis*), cypress (*Cupressus sempervirens*), fennel (*Foeniculum vulgare*), mint (*Mentha piperita*), pine (*Pinus sylvestris*), rose (*Rosa x centifolia*), and rosemary (*Rosmarinus officinalis*).

Essential oils and vegetable oils that appear in the photographs were supplied by NHR Organic Oils, Brighton, Sussex, UK BH1 5TN (www.nhrorganicoils.com), Oshadhi Organic and Wildcrafted Essential Oils, Cambridge, UK (www.oshadhi.co.uk), Tisserand Aromatherapy, West Sussex, UK BN6 9LS (www.tisserand.com), the Frankincense Store, London, UK NW1 8AH (www.freeyoursenses.co.uk), and

Base Formula Limited, Melton Mowbray, Leicestershire, UK LE13 0RG (www.baseformula.com). Please also note that when not being photographed or used, the essential oils featured are kept inside a closed container, which protects them from UV light, and are stored in a fridge to keep them cool.

My thanks to all of the authors and publishers whose works I quote in the following pages, including:

Page 2 (top) from *Revolution* by Russell Brand, published by Century; reproduced by permission of the Random House Group Ltd. © 2014

Page 2 (bottom), Vidyamala Burch, *Breathworks,* www.breathworks -mindfulness.org.uk

Pages 12 and 13–14, *Beyond Mindfulness in Plain English* by Bhante Henepola Gunaratana, © 2009 by Bhante Henepola Gunaratana; reprinted by permission of Wisdom Publications, www.wisdompubs .org.

Page 26, Prem Rawat, TimelessToday, www.timelesstoday.com

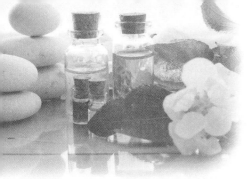

Introduction

*Coming into the Now with Mindfulness,
Meditation, and Essential Oils*

The stillest point of a seesaw is at its pivoting center.

MEDITATION AND MINDFULNESS

While there are various techniques and styles of meditation, all medi-tation appears to share the same universal objective: attainment of a state of inner calm and peace. The specific emphasis provided by the use of the term *mindfulness* or *mindful awareness* is that of defining the central aim as simply to *be,* to hone and sustain conscious awareness of *being* in the present moment.

Unconditional consciousness of the present moment naturally disables and dispels thoughts entrenched in the past or future. At the epicenter of the present moment, there is no place for past regrets, trau-mas, or disappointments; there is also no place for future fears, joyful anticipations, uncertainty, or expectations. They do not exist. In real-ity, we actually only ever exist in the present moment. This is reflected across many disciplines, as described by actor, activist, and proponent of Transcendental Meditation Russell Brand:

I shall tell you now and for no extra charge that "living in the present" seems to be the key component across every scripture, self-help book and religious group I've encountered. To harmonize with life in each moment, not to make happiness contingent on any prospective condition. Not to be tormented by the past but to live in the reality of "now," all else being mental construct.[1]

Conscious of being in the immediacy of now, we are more awake to our experience of the world, the environment around us, and our immediate inner and outer senses. Sustaining present moment consciousness through mindfulness or meditation is like bringing color to a sepia picture, switching on a light, or pulling back a curtain from a window. Moment-centered consciousness allows us to clearly see, experience, and sensually observe the richness of what is actually here and now. This is "en-lightenment." Darkness is not the opposite of light but the absence of light; it therefore cannot exist where there is light. Objects blocking light create a shadow, and once they are removed, the shadow no longer exists.

Ruminating thoughts, memories of the past, concerns for the future, or present worries, such as about an unpaid bill, may insidiously move into the foreground of awareness, filling the frame of consciousness and creating shadows. Meditation enables the perceiver to reevaluate the pictures that arise, allowing awareness to encompass the whole scene unimpeded, not just the objects that have come to occupy center stage.

Meditation/mindfulness is a proactive, conscious choice, a gentle process the perceiver may apply:

The emphasis on present moment awareness recognizes that this moment is the only moment in which we can act: past moments are only memories that we cannot change directly and future moments are only ideas. But with a realistic appraisal of thoughts, emotions and bodily sensations as they are perceived in the present moment we can move from a passive reactive mode of behavior to one that is infused with initiative and choice.[2]

Meditation is a voluntary process that is safe and cost-effective. More significantly, it offers a tool that potentially supports individuals in maintaining their personal locus of control, without the unwelcome side effects often associated with taking antidepressant or sedative drugs (although these do, in some instances, play an important role as temporary support). Where drug medication is unavoidably necessary, the concurrent practice of meditation, in some circumstances, has been shown to reduce the quantity required and the duration of their prescription.

THE COMPLEMENTARY ROLE OF ESSENTIAL OILS

Essential oils have accompanied us like guardians and companions on our ever-evolving journey through time and life, appearing in the form of fumigants, incense, cleansers, antiseptics, antibiotics, bactericides, and preservatives, as well as psychosomatic, hedonistic perfumes, which have not only been worn to adorn and attract but also to protect, to symbolize intention, and to punctuate and accentuate rite and ritual.

Modern scientific investigation, equipment, and methodology have enabled greater insight into the practical mechanisms, properties, components, and chemistry of organic and inorganic matter, providing better understanding of the world around us. They have also taught us much about the physical body and its healthy function, as well as about viruses, bacteria, disease, and the significant role diet and lifestyle (as well as attitude) play in supporting and maintaining wellness. As holistic health and well-being resurges into the foreground, so too the mind-body-spirit connection is increasingly recognized and acknowledged as a significant feature of wellness.

Essential oils continue to be used—as they have been throughout history—for their protective, restorative, rehabilitative, hedonistic qualities, seamlessly providing physiological and psycho-emotional-spiritual support, apparently bridging the pragmatic, natural, and ethereal dynamics of life and existence. In this respect, rather than separating one view from another (reductionism vs. vitalism), science may contribute, dispelling misguided myth and misbelief, providing insight into the amazing capacity of the body, and confirming the complementary relationship and role that plants, energetic medicines, and remedies play in assisting maintenance of health and homeostatic balance—the best of both worlds. Indeed, applied as medicine, as beautifying ingredients, and as spiritual aids, the unifying quality of essential oils provides a link between humans, nature, and psycho-spiritual realms.

Numerous references are made within historical medical texts, treatises, and scriptures demonstrating this dynamic role:

> He who has two cakes of bread, let him dispose of one of them for some flowers of the narcissus; for bread is the food of the body, and the narcissus is the food of the soul.
>
> GALEN (129–200 CE), GREEK PHYSICIAN,
> SURGEON, AND PHILOSOPHER

> The sick man . . . thou shalt place . . .
> Thou shalt cover his face
> Burn cypress and herbs . . .
> That the great gods may remove the evil
> That the evil spirit may stand aside
> . . .
> May a kindly spirit, a kindly genius be present.
>
> ANCIENT BABYLONIAN
> INCANTATION FOR FEVER,
> ASAKKI MARSUTI, TABLET XI[3]

> Before the dress is resumed, oils or ointments are rubbed in, and fragrant powders sprinkled on the skin.
>
> AVICENNA (980–1037 CE), THE CANON OF MEDICINE[4]

The herbs ought to be distilled when they are in their greatest vigor, and so ought the Flowers also.

NICHOLAS CULPEPER (1616–1654),
THE ENGLISH PHYSITIAN ENLARGED[5]

Then the Lord said to Moses, "Take fragrant spices—gum resin, onycha and galbanum—and pure frankincense, all in equal amounts, and make a fragrant blend of incense, the work of the perfumer."

EXODUS 30:34[6]

Perfume and incense bring joy to the heart.

PROVERBS 27:9

The smoke of the incense, together with the prayers of God's people, went up before God from the angel's hand.

REVELATIONS 8:4

Lord Krishna states that He enters into every particle of earth with His energy, prevailing over all the Earth with His prowess and supports all moving and non-moving *jivas* or embodied beings. He, Himself, is the luminosity of moonlight which nourishes all herbs and crops such as rice, fruits and grains.

SRIMAD BHAGAVAD-GITA 15:13[7]

Your plants are an orchard of pomegranates with choice fruits, with henna and nard, nard and saffron, calamus and cinnamon, with every kind of incense tree, with myrrh and aloes and all the finest spices. You are a garden fountain, a well of flowing water streaming down from Lebanon.

SONG OF SOLOMON 4:13–15

Evidenced through their historic and continued use in religious, cultural, and spiritual practices, essential oils significantly provide qualities potentially supportive in the context of prayer, intentional focus, and meditation. They have a demonstrated psycho-emotional influence on the limbic system, variously affecting mood and emotion, with the capacity to calm, sedate, or uplift. Certain essential oils, such as frankincense and patchouli, regulate breathing, instilling a sense of peace and tranquility; they consequently aid in quieting an anxious, racing mind. Other essential oils, such as rose and mandarin, are gently stimulating and uplifting. Yet others, among them lavender and geranium, possess both calming and stimulating qualities and are emotionally balancing.

Essential oils also have the ability to anchor us in our experience of the moment through the immediacy of fragrance awareness, especially when they are deliberately directly inhaled (drops on a tissue, for example) or infused into the surrounding environment.

Indeed, odor detection forms an ancient, intrinsic facet of human (and animal) survival mechanisms and is powerfully associated with memory. Thus, essential oils can be applied to reinforce memory and to aid recall of events, thoughts, and feelings experienced during original odor detection, as well as instilling or procuring attributed psycho-emotional qualities. For example, an essential oil or blend of essential oils diffused and detected during meditation may be deliberately inhaled afterward to trigger recollection of the experience of being in meditation, thus potentially recapturing the sense of stillness and calmness felt there and then in the here and now. This can act as a reminder to continue to meditate, to maintain conscious awareness of the present moment, and to experience feelings of calm and peace here and now.

This facet, along with their other significant psycho-emotional qualities, renders essential oils valuable complementary tools, particularly when applied with techniques such as counseling, psychotherapy, and cognitive behavioral therapy (CBT), as well as meditation and relaxation techniques.

Essential oils are effective when used individually, but their effects may potentially increase when they are carefully blended together. As well

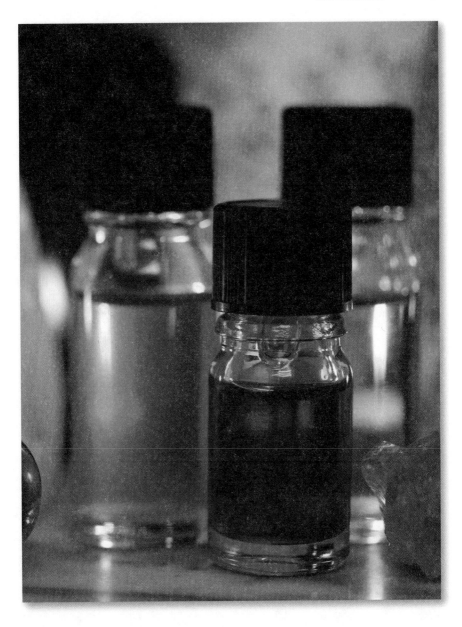

as their chemical and therapeutic properties, the sensual, fragrant qualities of essential oils lend pleasure and expressive creativity to the art of blending.[8] So in this sense scent, like color, can be applied to paint a picture, create ambience, and express and enhance feelings, emotions, and moods, while at the same time providing valuable immunological support.

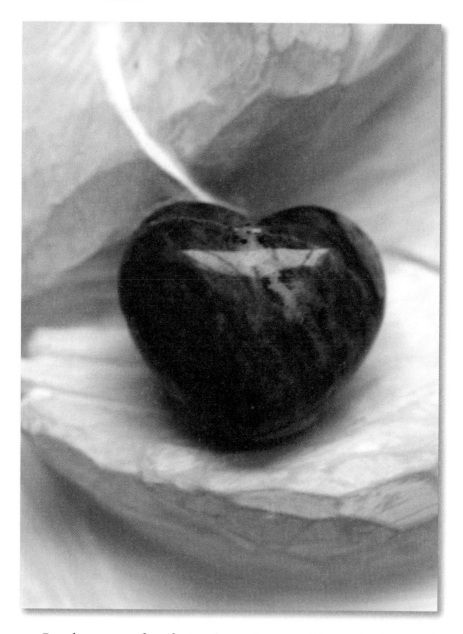

Based on years of professional experience working with clients and students, this book offers an introductory yet informative self-help guide that will support the practical and safe use of essential oils as a complement to mindfulness and meditation.

Chapter 1 of this book will introduce you to both the theory and practice of mindfulness, identifying the types of practices that mindful-ness includes, with enough instruction to guide you to practice, along with some indications of the research supporting the benefits of these practices and some personal reflections on meditation.

Chapter 2 offers a clear basic description of essential oil chemistry and how various oils interact with our psychosomatic systems. There are hundreds of essential oils available to purchase over the counter or through mail order. However, not all are suitable for personal use. Essential oils are mainly produced for the pharmaceutical, food and manufacturing, perfume, and cosmetics industries. Indeed, the aroma-therapy market accounts for less than 5 percent of the total overall quantity of essential oils produced. Chapter 2 will guide you through the copious offerings to make your own selections and learn the various means of safely using and applying essential oils.

A select but significant complementary group of essential oils is highlighted in chapter 2 to provide a foundation on which to build your repertoire. This specific group of essential oils was originally purposefully derived to apply in the context of special needs (work-ing with vulnerable or sensitive clients) and includes some of the potentially least hazardous (although no essential oil is completely hazard-free) yet still very effective essences. Collectively referred to as Serenity Essential Oils, they cover a valuable spectrum of therapeutic properties pertinent for those wishing to use essential oils as self-help remedies and for the discerning student to apply as a sound founda-tion for learning.

In order to help contextualize their properties, however, the infor-mation presented here includes a wide range of essential oils. Serenity Essential Oils are highlighted among these for ease of identification and are covered in most depth. Essential oils that possess qualities particu-larly pertinent to meditation and relaxation are described, with easy-to-follow charts to help you identify their properties and assist and guide your selection.

Chapter 3 covers the major means of applying essential oils for personal use, providing sufficient detail for you to make your own preparations, including creams, lotions, and ointments, as well as inhalers and diffusers.

In addition to mindfulness and essential oils, wellness is enhanced by the addition of relaxation techniques, sufficient exercise, and healthy nutrition. Chapter 4 provides a schematic overview of these important tools.

A bibliography of recommended resources is also supplied, making this book a guide well suited to offer you the means to fully enter into the serenity, creativity, and wholesomeness of each fragrant moment of now.

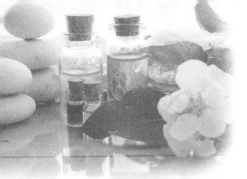

1

What Is Mindfulness?

Why and How to Make It Part of Your Life

Mindfulness is a state of consciously being aware, of paying attention to and maintaining concentration on and consciousness of the here and now. It is *being* in the present moment, noticing what is happening internally and externally without pre-judgment, condition, or expectation, but with gentle acceptance, unconditional intentionality, and equanimity (calmness of temper, composure). In *Mindfulness and Mental Health,* a cogent summary of the field, author and psychotherapist Chris Mace clarifies:

> Mindfulness is a way of being aware—mindful awareness is receptive not exclusive. Sensations, thoughts or feelings are simply experienced for what they are. To be mindfully aware means, strangely, there can be no "mind." Even if thoughts are chattering away, they receive no more attention than anything else that has arisen. As people's ordinary, reactive ways of restricting their awareness diminishes, a sense of the suchness of things emerges.[1]

An aspect of insight meditation, mindfulness evolved from Buddhism and was introduced to the West during the 1970s. Although steeped in Buddhist philosophy, the simplicity of its processes and practice enables its presentation in nonreligious, independent contexts as an aid to focus attention on the here and now: conscious, present-centered awareness amidst the rhythm of daily life. In hospitals and in clinical practice, mindfulness has demonstrated some success in alleviating the experience of depression, anxiety, post-traumatic stress disorder, stress, and stress-related conditions, so it is often recommended as a supportive self-help technique. It has also been included in management of chronic pain.

In his extensive writings about mindfulness, Buddhist monk Bhante Henepola Gunaratana explains that it is not necessary to be a Buddhist to benefit:

> So, how much faith do you need? Do you need to convert to Buddhism? Do you need to abandon the tradition in which you were raised or the ideals to which you have deep commitment? Do you need to set aside anything that your intellect or understanding of the world tells you? Absolutely not. You can retain your current frame of reference and accept only what you are prepared to accept, a piece at a time, and only what you in fact find helpful. Yet you do need *some* faith. You need the same kind of faith that you need to read a good novel or conduct a scientific experiment. You need "a willing suspension of disbelief" . . . faith, which at heart is nothing more than the willingness to accept provisionally something without yet having proved or verified it for oneself.[2]

Meditation per se is an experiential process that apparently provides a bridge between the finite and infinite (or the deepest sense of inner being). In this sense the meditator may evolve through various phases, or layers, of consciousness, from physical finite awareness to states of deep, wordless inner awareness, enlightening realization, and deep understanding. In *Holistic Consciousness,* author, mystic, and theological scholar Phiroz Mehta details *wordless* in this way: "not conveyed or perceived as idea or thought in our ordinary meaning of those words but as immediate, direct, shapeless and formless realization in and by holistic consciousness . . . later [given] shape and form as inspired idea and word."[3]

In a 2004 article, "Coming to Our Senses," Jon Kabat-Zinn, one of the foremost exponents of mindfulness-based stress reduction (MBSR), observes the "miracle of the five senses" as tools that ground and anchor and enable access to full awareness and appreciation of the moment experience, "seeing that which is here to be seen, hearing that which is here to be heard, etc.—the five senses plus what the Buddha included as the sixth and most important and unifying sense, which is the capacity of the mind itself for non-conceptual knowing."[4]

The techniques of mindful attention take the perceiver to the well but the techniques are not the water. The water (experience) drawn from the well and contained within the cup (mindful attention) offers a taste, an insight, of the ocean. The techniques of meditation, or concentrated focus, can be seen as the cup that enables the perceiver to draw from the inner depths of the well awareness of innate and infinite spirit within (not outside, above, or beyond, but inside and available).

Mindful (or intentional) awareness practice and *deep concentration meditation* are two modes of mindfulness practice.

MINDFUL AWARENESS PRACTICE

The practice of mindful or intentional awareness (*vipassana*) focuses on being awake to what is happening in the immediacy of here and now, noticing what is being felt, observed, or experienced in any given moment, internally and externally. As Gunaratana explains, this is achieved by employing the mind to check focused attention:

Clear comprehension means remaining fully awake and conscious in the midst of any activity, everything your body is doing and everything you are perceiving. It is a turned-within monitoring of everything going on in the mind and body. Clear comprehension requires "bare attention" ("bare" in the sense of stripped down or nothing added over the top) to assure that you are mindful of the right things and mindful in the right way. It is a quality control factor that monitors what is being noticed and how the noticing is taking place.[5]

Being aware in the moment and holding that awareness by anchoring to the immediacy of what is felt, sensed, and observed, internally and externally, brings the perceiver to the gateway of conscious awareness, of simply being. Practicing mindful awareness enables a focusing of attention on the here and now. Simply *being* within the moment experience potentially instills a sense of peace, completeness, and acceptance (among other qualities)—a wordless sense of the fullness of existence.

So, to elaborate, here and now I am sitting at my table with my hands poised on the keyboard of my laptop. I feel the breeze entering the barge through the open window brushing against my face as I concentrate on typing these words. I hear a distant duck quacking, the sound of the wind blowing against the half-open window shutter, rustling the leaves in the trees outside, and the cars in the distance humming. I notice the fading light around me as the sun sets outside, and the birds twittering; I notice that my neck and shoulders are aching from holding the same position for too long. I notice the bitter, pungent taste in my mouth of the coffee I drank a moment ago, its flavor still on my breath. I feel the pressure of the chair against my bottom and my feet on the soft rug lying across the solid wooden floor. As I focus on these immediate sensations (albeit in scattered observation), I am aware that I feel peaceful. I notice I am conscious of my breathing and feel the softness and warmth of the air as it passes through my nose into my throat, warmly filling my lungs, then rising and exiting down my nose. In this moment my sense of peace is comforting and filling. Using the immediacy of this sensual check, I am brought to the gate of conscious awareness, and in this state of conscious awareness I find myself in peace.

I can do this as an exercise, following a less scattered, prescribed routine of noticing, perhaps as a body scan. Or I can find a starting point and then allow my experience to emerge as I focus attention on a selected object or point within my vision, holding the object in steady view while allowing my consciousness, my vision, to remain open to the whole peripheral territory, noticing at the same time what I feel inside, in my body, my rambling thoughts, my physical sensations; there is no resistance but observation, acknowledgment, and acceptance.

I can practice this focused attention at times during the day, to anchor myself to the moment, to hone my awareness to the present, as I find myself distracted and drawn into events around me, noticing as I eat my food, wash the dishes, walk to the car, and sit in discourse with my students. I can give "bare attention," unconditional and nonjudgmental.

Mindful or intentional awareness practice is *a way of being,* a moment-to-moment experience best appreciated through regular, daily attention, compassionate self-discipline, and tenacity. The impact is more fully appreciated when practice is frequent and regular—little and often rather than once a week or every so often. Intentional awareness precedes deeper meditative states; thus the consequence of mindfulness may extend beyond merely providing a coping strategy or relaxation technique to apply during stressful periods of life. Crisis often acts as a catalyst for change, however. The experiential process of adopting mindful awareness and meditation as a coping tool may consequently lead to enlightened discovery of an awareness of presence and being not previously considered, or overlooked, as professor of psychology Shauna L. Shapiro and associates acknowledge: "Formal meditation seeps into daily life, bringing greater nonjudgmental consciousness to everything that one does, feels and experiences."[6]

Focus on present awareness, on being in the moment, is also applied as a tool in gestalt therapy, cognitive behavioral therapy (CBT), and counseling. Psychologist and humanistic philosopher Erich Fromm, for example, in his book *The Art of Listening,* pertinently observes: "It is important to see the patient [client] as the hero of a drama and not to see him [or her] as a summation of complexes. And, actually, every human being is the hero of a drama."[7] Seeing, feeling, sensing, becoming aware enables clarity, which in turn facilitates mobilization of energy to do something, to become consciously proactive; energy becomes focused, deliberately directed, and thus more effective.

This perspective holds true for and encapsulates the essence of most helping professions, particularly integrative therapies such as acupuncture, essential oil therapy, Bowen, yoga, the cognitive therapies mentioned above, and mindful awareness and practice. Significantly, Fromm acknowledges, "Mindfulness means awareness. I am fully aware at every moment of my body, including my posture, anything that goes on in my body, and I am fully aware of my thoughts, of what I think; I am fully concentrated."[8]

Thus, mindful awareness practice is incorporated intentionally to anchor a client (or individual) into their present moment experience, which can be especially pertinent when working with conditions such as anxiety, depression, and post-traumatic stress disorder (PTSD), where a grounded sense of the present, a point to start at and return to in cyclical exploratory journeying and closure, is significant. Carl Rogers, father of client-centered therapy, reiterates this, relating the significance of the counselor being present and aware in a conscious state of acceptance that is underpinned by the condition of being in congruence, positive regard, and empathy. Counselors seek to maintain awareness and attention while they "walk alongside their client" in the present moment: "When we provide a psychological climate that permits a person to *be* . . . we are tapping into a tendency which permeates all organic life."[9]

DEEP CONCENTRATION MEDITATION

Deep concentration meditation (*shamatha*) is the second mode of mindfulness (although some prefer to refer to it as "gentle awareness" rather than "deep concentration" to accentuate the sense of choice

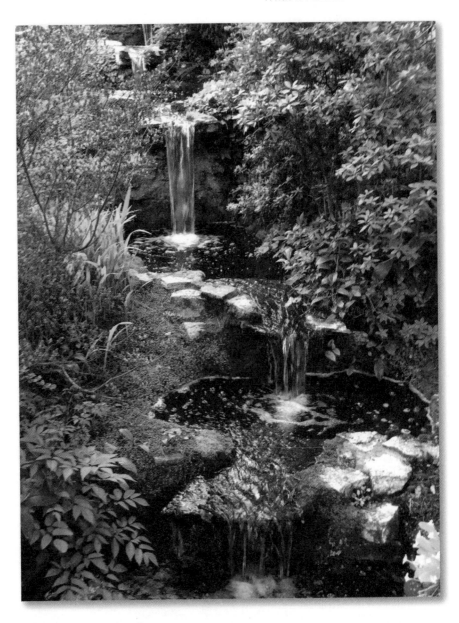

underpinning this practice). Mindfulness awareness practice helps lay the groundwork for deeper meditation, which focuses concentration more specifically. Gentle self-discipline is applied to hone focus and concentration. This deeper concentration meditation has four specific foundations:

1. Mindfulness of the body
2. Mindfulness of feelings
3. Mindfulness of consciousness
4. Mindfulness of mental objects

These four foundational pillars provide the cornerstones of the Noble Eightfold Path. Just as in the proverbial "elephant and the blind men" (each feeling a different part of the elephant—the trunk, the foot, the ear, the tail—and proclaiming the elephant to be a snake or a drum and so on), there is some variance in the language selected by different authors to depict these qualities, demonstrated in the following table, which first compares the Noble Eightfold Path as described by Bhante Gunaratana[10] and by Mace.[11] Second, it compares the qualities of mindfulness as listed by positive psychologists Snyder and Lopez[12] with those listed by Shapiro et al.[13]

THE ESSENTIAL THEMES AND QUALITIES OF MINDFULNESS PRACTICE AND MEDITATION

THE NOBLE EIGHTFOLD PATH	
GUNARATANA (2009)	**MACE (2008)**
1. Right view	1. Morality (sita)
2. Right resolve	2. Concentration (samadhi)
3. Right speech	3. Wisdom (panna)
4. Right action	**The factors that make for concentration are:**
5. Right livelihood	1. Right effort
6. Right effort	2. Right awareness
7. Right mindfulness	3. Right concentration
8. Right concentration	4. Right understanding
	5. Right thought
	Three essential interdependent characteristics of *being* are:
	1. Unsatisfactoriness suffering (dukka)
	2. Transience (anicca)
	3. Absence of self (annatta)

MINDFULNESS QUALITIES	
SNYDER AND LOPEZ (2007)	**SHAPIRO ET AL. (2005)**
Acceptance	Loving kindness
Empathy	Nonjudgment
Generosity	Nonstriving
Gentleness	Openness
Gratitude	Patience
Letting go	Trust

In spite of variance in the descriptive language, the overarching core themes emanating from the above appear to provide a general formula for *correct behavior* and *attitude (moral conduct), right concentration,* and *right mindfulness (right wisdom).* The outcome of this, as Gunaratana expresses, is "bright wakefulness,"[14] or, as Shapiro et al. suggest, the intention behind meditation is to wake up from this suboptimal state (or "normality" or "developmental arrest") of consciousness, to wake up to our true nature.[15] The reward of mindful awareness and meditation is an enriched, deeper experiential spiritual knowing or the sense of simply "what is."

MINDFULNESS MEDITATION PRACTICE

Even though steeped in Buddhist philosophy, mindfulness meditation practice is not intended to be *religious* (although there is inevitably an element of spirituality). Practice requires consistency but not obsession, rite, or ritual. Although sometimes rite and ritual act as reminders that may superficially assist practice, it is important to remember that there is a difference between discipline and obsession. Advocates of this process suggest that mindful awareness practice and meditation may coexist with other beliefs or may be used and practiced independent of any belief. Mindfulness is a practical, simple process that merely supports concentration on the here and now and the experience of simply being.

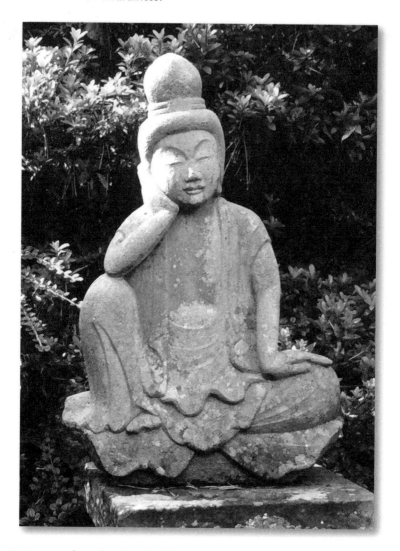

It is true, though, that the "temporary suspension of disbelief" mentioned by Gunaratana appears to require a certain amount of faith, held at least long enough to allow the consequential experience of mindfulness practice to manifest, especially as this is not always immediately obvious. Only through continual gentle practice do the consequential effects begin to emerge into the foreground of conscious awareness, seeping into daily life, bringing greater consciousness to "everything that one does, feels and experiences."[16]

Sakyong Mipham Rinpoche, head of the Tibetan Shambhala

lineage, blends Eastern and Western perspectives within his teachings. He recommends meditating for ten to twenty minutes twice a day in a place that is not too noisy or distracting, sitting cross-legged or on a chair with feet touching the ground, holding or supporting a straight back, then gazing a few inches in front of the face, eyes lowered, focusing on an object or the breath or both.[17] Peripheral vision is not embraced beyond the object of gazing. Holding the gaze, the mind is gently brought back from wandering to the object of focus or the breath, which is gentle and unforced. The intention is to achieve peace of mind and compassionate awareness, and to allow this condition of awareness to permeate to consciousness of being.

The subtle simplicity of mindfulness, however, does raise academic debate, especially as even among the various Buddhist traditions there is variance in descriptive terms, as identified above (for example, concentration versus gentle awareness). In a 2009 article in *Clinical Psychology Review,* Chambers and associates question whether "mindfulness represents a distinct construct or a quality of consciousness that spans and incorporates other states,"[18] identifying two potential dimensions to mindfulness practice: pre-thought present moment experience and secondary processing, where thought-awareness (or cognitive interpretation) identifies conditions such as acceptance and nonjudgment, thus deviating from the condition of complete pre-thought, present-centered, *nonjudgmental* awareness.

This disparity equally lends itself to the interpretational perspective (spiritual, religious, and personal values) of the authors, the deliverers (teachers or guides), and the receivers (students, clients, or readers). Evaluative description, for example, is conveyed through the lens (and language) of the experiencer's own relationship with the process (again, the elephant and the blind men). This slant may potentially influence expression and formulation of prescribed practical processes and the description and portrayal of information. Somehow the *just being* element becomes shrouded or obscured, even lost (perhaps like when trying to grasp a slippery piece of soap), in trying to emotionally and cognitively *understand*, *justify*, and *describe* the process, to attempt to tangibly make sense of its practice and experience.

To avoid this ambiguity and confusion, Gunaratana recommends that it is better to say what mindfulness *does* rather than trying to explain what it *is*.[19] For example, the practice of mindfulness, as with any meditation technique, initially involves tangible and practical processes, such as the act of focusing on an object, and the *outcome* of practicing meditation is observable, comparable, and measurable, such as improved concentration, calmness, and equanimity.

WHAT MINDFULNESS *DOES*: RESEARCH EVIDENCE

In "Meditation and Positive Psychology," Shapiro and associates acknowledge that Buddhist theory and mindfulness appear to complement and share some affinity with psychology, especially the quality of encouraging positive personal self-awareness. They suggest that "meditation provides road maps to reach optimal openness, awareness and insight."[20] Mace, for example, reported on a study on meditation and psychotherapy conducted by Kutz et al. of twenty patients using mindfulness alongside psychotherapy, in which they observed an overall reduction in negativity and anxiety (although they also observed that hostility, relationships, family and sexual adjustment, and emotional inhibition generally appeared unaffected).[21] Significantly, Kutz et al. noted some change through the course of meditation involving capacity to access feelings and memories that had not been visited for years, improvements in insight, and the capacity to continue to use therapy productively, suggesting these traits do indicate the viable, cost-effective potential of integrating mindfulness practice alongside other therapeutic approaches.[22]

In a 2009 study published in the *Journal of Cognitive Psychotherapy* that examined the effects of mindfulness-based stress reduction (MBSR) on the brain behavior mechanism of self-referential processing in fourteen patients with social anxiety disorder, researchers observed increased self-esteem and decreased anxiety, increased positive and decreased negative self-endorsement, increased activity in areas of the brain related to attention regulation, and reduced activity in brain systems implicated in conceptual-linguistic self-view.[23] They suggest the practice of MBSR techniques may have a positive influence on maladjusted or distorted social self-view, potentially related to changes in the way people view themselves and their ability to maintain attention. This is explained as a result of positively rephrasing internal dialogue and consciously breaking the habit of internal negative narrative. Regularly engaging in mindfulness practice actually altered neural pathways and areas of activity within the brain, ultimately reprogramming self-defeating tendencies and dialogue that reinforced negative behavior, thus providing capacity for and enabling positive self-perspective.

In a study published in *Applied Nursing Research* in 2006 researchers found that nurses and nurses aides, recruited from long-term complex continuing care units in a large geriatric teaching hospital in America, and engaged in a program of mindfulness practice, experienced significant improvements in burnout symptoms, relaxation, and life satisfaction compared with a control group.[24] Consequently, their recommendation was that mindfulness practice offered a promising method of managing stress among staff. Similarly, Shapiro and associates, in a 2005 study involving health-care professionals (nurses, social workers, physiotherapists, and psychologists) who participated in a MBSR program, reported decrease in perceived stress and greater self-compassion when compared with controls (compassion is encapsulated in the list of mindful qualities above).[25] Reported psychological distress, dissatisfaction with life, and job burnout were also decreased, although the differences between the experimental and the control groups were not significant in this respect. However, participants did indicate that the MBSR program had a substantially positive impact on their lives. The authors did report a significantly higher than average dropout rate (44%); dropout participants attributed their departure from the program to difficulty in managing their workload as well as being involved in the study, especially in view of the limited time available to them!

Wang et al., in their 2010 paper published in *Psychiatry Research,* found that the frontal regions, anterior cingulate cortex, limbic system, and parietal lobes within the brain were affected during meditative states, noting strong correlations between depth of meditation and neural activity in the left inferior forebrain relating to the subjective experience of the meditators.[26] In the same journal, in 2011, Holzel published results of a study that examined the neural effect of an MBSR program on sixteen healthy, meditation-naive participants and observed increases in gray matter concentration within the left hippocampus.[27] Whole brain analysis identified increases in the posterior cingulate cortex, the temporo-parietal junction, and the cerebellum in the MBSR group compared with the controls, indicating changes in brain regions involved in learning and memory process, emotion regulation, self-referential processing, and perspective taking. Goldin et al., supporting this result, identified positive correlation between brain activity in the prefrontal region of the brain from neuro-images taken of patients with social anxiety disorder before and during mindfulness appraisal; MBSR resulted in moderate reduction of symptoms of social anxiety, depression, ruminating thoughts, and states of anxiety and increased self-esteem.[28]

Such results confirm the potential to positively change or reprogram neural mechanisms through mindfulness practice. Engaging in regular practice of meditation appears to have a calming effect, which may permeate beyond the duration and state of being in meditation. Negative self-defeating narrative and thought patterns, attitude, perception, and behavior may be reversed or improved through being suspended in the *experience of being* in a positive, unthreatened state during meditation, and through deliberate positive internal affirmation, retraining or retuning neural pathways. This positive sense of being whole and complete irrespective of the condition (anxiety, depression, ruminating thoughts, physical pain), being consciously calm and self-approving through employing the mindful qualities of kindness and compassion, enables a person to identify their true locus of control. Thus the present-centered quality of mindfulness does appear effective in alleviating anxiety and supporting improved self-image and perception. Anchoring the perceiver to their present moment experience paradoxically also appears to instigate a journey of renewed self-discovery.

Research evidence examining brain images during the process of meditation demonstrates significant consequential neural response, indicating that regular meditation practice aids in positive restructuring of negative self-narrative, thoughts, attitudes, and behaviors in a way that enhances self-compassion and positive self-image and reduces feelings of anxiety, depression, and ruminating thoughts. Essential oils stimulate and influence similar neural pathways and areas within the brain, thus sharing some affinity with the practice of meditation, particularly when considering their ability to sedate, calm, ground, and uplift the recipient. However, largely due to a lack of funding, there is limited or no similar brain-imaging research evidence available to verify (or disprove) this affinity to date.

PERSONAL REFLECTION

Having practiced meditation for more than forty years (although duration or length of time in the context of meditation is not relevant, as it is always a present moment experience), I recognize many of the elements described in the literature regarding the experience of mindful awareness practice and meditation. I was taught Prem Rawat's meditation, which focuses on techniques that hone attention inwardly and, like mindfulness, is not attached to a specific religion. Consciousness of being in the moment is a shared significant feature, as is the ability to surrender, let go, and allow consciousness of the experience of meditating to permeate awareness. This meditation is also very simple. The only condition is the regular practice of the meditation techniques;

there is no doctrine. As with mindfulness, it is an experiential process; only proactive engagement in it yields the consequential appreciation and feeling of connectedness and peace. As Prem Rawat expressed it: "Peace needs to be in everyone's life. It is not the world that needs peace, it is people. When people in the world are at peace within, the world will be at peace. The peace that we are looking for is within. It is in the heart, waiting to be felt."[29]

When I practice mindful awareness, it is automatically, seamlessly accompanied by my conscious awareness of the meditation breathing technique I have practiced for years; one seems to enhance the other. Indeed, breath focus features in all meditative processes and techniques of relaxation. However, in some instances, breath focus is undesirable (for example, during anxiety and panic attacks or in obsessive compulsive disorder), as focused attention on breathing can exacerbate a tendency for overbreathing, panic, or an obsessive need to control. Or it may remind a person of previous experiences of being in negative states and so trigger a similar response (mental distraction from being overfocused is best employed in these circumstances). Concentration on meditation is not forced or rigid but gentle, achieved through compassionate awareness, rather than military-like prescription, discipline, obsession, and regime.

I find the practice of mindful awareness useful in preparing myself prior to and ending formal meditation. I also practice mindful awareness intermittently during the day. I am not always in a state of mindful awareness or meditation, but I do have a choice; in returning my attention to either, I am aware that whatever I am concentrating on, my experience of *being* is always constantly, conditionlessly there. I find the techniques of mindful awareness a practical, tangible construct. Deliberately noticing and paying attention to internal and external sensations and experience does provide a road map,[30] a point of reference to direct my awareness toward my own moment-focus, reminding me to remain in a state of centered consciousness.

I also notice that if I diffuse an essential oil or blend of essential oils during the formal process of meditation, I am able to recall the experience of calmness felt if I smell this fragrance later in the day as I attend to other things. This in turn inspires or reminds me to remain aware of being in the moment, to hold the sense of calmness and awareness of "there and then" renewed in the "here and now." Remaining conscious of *being* in the present moment, I am at the gateway, the bridge, between finite and infinite awareness. Holding, with compassion, this awareness of *being here and now* dissolves the veil of separation.

Some argue, however, that concerted focus on the moment may also

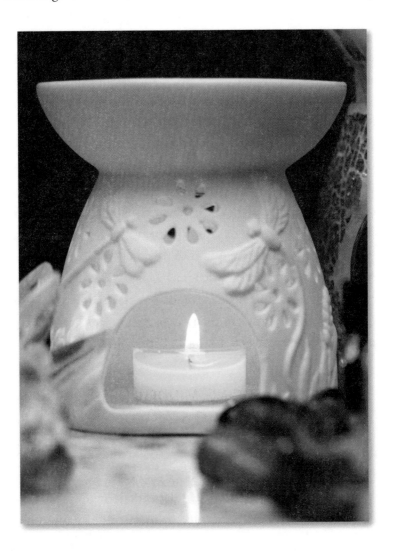

draw unwelcome attention to or intensify those thoughts or feelings occupying the immediate frame of awareness, as if honing attention appears to consent to their place at center stage so they seem even more pronounced. It is true, and I speak from personal experience, that for this reason there are times when meditation is not desirable. In such circumstances where unpleasant thoughts, memories, emotional feelings, or pain are extremely loud or overfocused, I find deliberate distraction through some other positive activity—physical action or mental concentration such as exercise, walking, painting, reading, watching an enthralling play or film, enjoying the company of good friends, setting a positive itinerary to follow—that absorbs my attention provides a more appropriate temporary tool. Purposefully drawing attention away from the intensity thus allows me to step aside for a moment. My perspective then is able to naturally dissipate more appropriately into context to calm the exaggerated loudness or brightness.

Of course, sometimes the object filling my awareness is there because it does need my attention (hunger, thirst, pain, and even the unpaid bill require expedient action). Also, it is possible that distraction can insidiously become, or can be deliberately applied to be, avoidant or denying, a cloak that shrouds from the pain, the fear, or whatever the issue is. Such distraction may appear to shield us from the pain and hurt that we believe and fear acknowledgment may expose us to. Sometimes a person requires support, assistance, or professional help too. In such circumstances meditation can be used as a complementary tool, when and if we are ready to accept the onus of control.

PRACTICING MINDFULNESS:
GETTING STARTED

Traditionally, prescribed "mindfulness stress reduction programs" run in eight-week blocks and generally consist of one- to two-hour sessions once a week and daily one-hour independent meditation practice. Having thus established a pattern or habit of mindful awareness and meditation, the attendee is equipped to continue independently. Rinpoche recommends meditating twice a day (morning and evening), in ten- to twenty-minute sessions (with compassionate acceptance if this routine is broken through other more immediate needs and demands—that is, being self-disciplined rather than obsessional). He recommends initially focusing on one of the following:

Initial Pre-meditation Mindfulness Focus

Yoga: Stretches and postures designed to enhance greater awareness of and to balance and strengthen the musculoskeletal system.

Body scan: Progressively moving attention from the toes to the head (or head to toes), observing any sensations in the different regions of the body.

Mindful awareness practice: Focusing on an object and the breath and the peripheral environment/noticing what is happening in the present moment (seeing/hearing/sensing/tasting/feeling/touching/walking/sitting/preparing food/getting dressed etc.).[31]

Sitting in Meditation

Holding gentle focus on an object. Being aware of body sensations, thoughts, and emotions while continually returning the focus of attention to the breath or returning attention to the object and immediate sensual awareness when the mind wanders.

In mindfulness, or shamatha, meditation, we are trying to achieve a mind that is stable and calm. What we begin to discover is that this calmness or harmony is a natural aspect of the mind. Through mindfulness practice we are just developing and strengthening it and eventually we are able to remain peacefully in our mind without struggling. Our mind naturally feels content.[32]

Being here and now in the rich stillness of the moment.

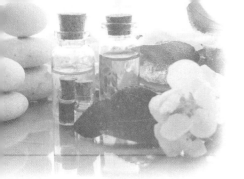

2

Essential Oils as Meditation Companions

The Science of Their Use

Essential oils possess numerous qualities that may support and enhance wellness and a sense of well-being. They may improve mental clarity and concentration. They may instill a sense of feeling calm and uplifted, energized, and awake. They are perfect meditation companions.

WHAT IS AN ESSENTIAL OIL?

Essential oils are highly concentrated, volatile, odiferous phytochemical derivatives extracted from various parts of certain plants, trees, and shrubs, such as rhizomes and roots, stems, leaves, flowering heads, seeds, wood (stumps, trunk, heartwood, sawdust), twigs, bark, resin, needles, berries, blossoms, fruit, rind, and grass.

Essential oil extraction mainly involves the process of steam distillation. The heat and pressure of steam forced through the plant material releases essential oils contained in secretory cells and glands. Citrus fruits, however, such as orange, mandarin, lemon, and grapefruit, are extracted by a process known as expression. This method involves crushing the fruit peel to squeeze out the essential oil held in secretory sacs. Citrus essential oils contain a high proportion of volatile terpene molecules, which are destroyed by intense heat.

Historically, essential oils were extracted by expression, or by maceration. Maceration involves steeping the plant material in warm animal fat, oil, or water. As the plant material becomes saturated, its structure breaks down, releasing the essential oils held within secretory cells. The oil, fat, or water mixture is strained to remove the plant material. The remaining essential oil–saturated substance is applied accordingly as a perfume, ointment (*anointment*), or healing salve.

Solvent extraction is similar to distillation; however, instead of water, or steam, a chemical substance (such as acetone, hexane, or toluene) is used to dissolve, encourage, or "soak out" volatile components. This method is less heat-intensive and is employed to remove essential oils from delicate plant materials such as petals and blossoms (for example, rose and jasmine) that would otherwise be destroyed by the heat and intense pressure of steam distillation. Solvent extraction produces a waxy concrete, which is then washed with a strong alcohol solution (such as ethanol) to remove as much of the wax as possible along with any remaining solvent. The alcohol is then dissolved by a method referred to as vacuum distillation, leaving behind a heavy, sticky resinoid known as an absolute. Absolutes contain solvent and alcohol residue and are not classified as *pure* essential oils. They are less volatile and, therefore, more tenacious than steam-distilled essential oils. The odor of an absolute is often quite intense. Absolutes are mainly used by the cosmetic and perfume industries as fixatives to prolong a fragrance.

A *pure* essential oil should present as it does at the point of distilled or expressed extraction, with nothing added or removed. Sometimes, however, it is necessary to redistill, or rectify, an essential oil to remove harmful molecules. For example, bergamot is rectified to remove the phototoxic furocoumarins and then labeled as bergamot FCF (furocoumarin-free).

EXAMPLES OF AREAS WHERE ESSENTIAL OILS ARE STORED WITHIN THE PLANT*

Bark	Cinnamon
Berries	Juniper
Blossoms	Neroli (orange blossom), *rose*, ylang ylang
Flowers	Calendula, *chamomile (German and Roman)*, clove bud, helichrysum, jasmine Flowering tops Clary sage, hyssop, *lavender*, lemon balm, marjoram, peppermint, rosemary, thyme
Fruits	Black pepper, May Chang, star anise
Grass (leaves)	Citronella, lemongrass, palmarosa
Leaves	*Cajeput*, cinnamon, clary sage, eucalyptus, hyssop, *lavender*, lemon balm, myrtle, niaouli, *patchouli*, peppermint, *petitgrain*, rosemary, sage, *tea tree*, thyme
Needles	*Cypress*, pine
Resins	*Frankincense, galbanum*, myrrh, tolu balsam
Rind	Bergamot, grapefruit, lemon, lime, *mandarin*, orange bitter
Roots, rhizomes	Angelica, ginger, *spikenard*, valerian, *vetivert*
Seeds	Bitter fennel, caraway, cardamom, *carrot seed*, coriander, fennel, nutmeg
Twigs and branches	*Cajeput*, cinnamon, *cypress*, eucalyptus, myrtle, niaouli, *petitgrain, tea tree*
Whole plant above ground	Bitter fennel, *geranium*, rosemary (poor quality), yarrow
Wood (stumps, trunk, heartwood, sawdust)	Cedarwood, rosewood, sandalwood

*The essential oils given in italics in this table are those oils I have specially selected and designated Serenity Essential Oils. Please see the next section for a full explanation.

Not all plants produce essential oils. According to Tisserand and Young, in their *Essential Oil Safety: A Guide for Health Professionals*,[1] and Brian M. Lawrence,[2] the eminent essential oil researcher and founder of the *Journal of Essential Oil Research*, there are an estimated

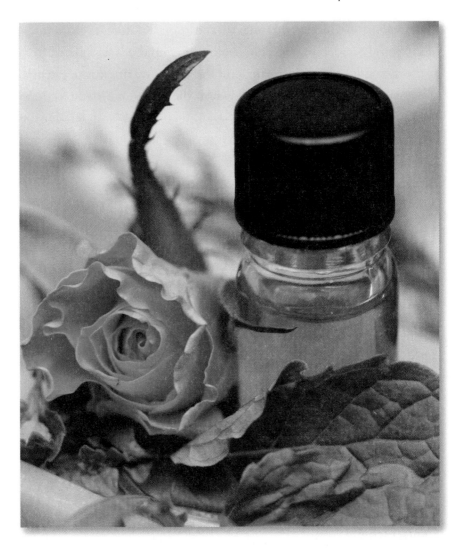

350,000 plant species existent throughout the world, of which just 17,500 (5%) are aromatic. Yet just 400 of these aromatic species surrender essential oils suitable for commercial use; 50 percent are specifically cultivated for their essential oil, while others are grown, managed, and harvested in the wild.

Essential oil–bearing plants mainly grow throughout the temperate forest, woodland, grassland, scrub, Mediterranean, and tropical forest climate regions. For example, German (blue) chamomile essential oil is sourced from plants growing in the northern European woodland and grass regions of Germany, Hungary, and the UK. Roman chamomile, along with lavender and other herbaceous essential oils, is sourced from plants growing in France, Spain, and the UK. The finest rose essential oil is sourced from rose bushes grown in the scrub and Mediterranean region of Turkey, Bulgaria, and Iran. Palmarosa and lemongrass are sourced from plants grown in the tropical regions of India and Guatemala. In some instances plants are grown in one region and distilled in another, for example in the case of dried spices.

Many essential oils are produced as a by-product of industry (for example, citrus oils such as orange, lemon, and lime are produced for the food, manufacturing, and perfume industries). The following list of the types of products and processed foods that contain essential oils illustrates the pervasiveness of these oils in our everyday lives.

Air fresheners

Alcohol

Animal feed

Antiseptics

Baked goods

Beverages (Earl Grey tea, jasmine and rose tea, herbal teas)

Candles

Confectionaries

Contact lenses

Convenience foods

Cosmetics and toiletries

Cough syrups

Dentistry products

Detergents

Disinfectants

Fabric conditioners

Food and drink flavorings

Food coloring

Gargles

Glue/adhesives

Ice cream

Insect repellents/insecticides

Lotions, creams

Meat products

Mouthwash

Nasal sprays

Ointments

Paint

Paper

Perfumes (eau-de-cologne, aftershave)

Pharmaceuticals (antibacterials, antifungals, decongestants)

Pizzas

Preservatives

Printing ink

Rubber manufacturing

Soap

Soap powder

Soft drinks

Stomach tonics/laxatives

Textiles

Throat lozenges

Tinned food

Tobacco

Toothpaste

Veterinary products

SERENITY ESSENTIAL OILS

Of the 400 aromatic species used as essential oils, I have designated fifteen as Serenity Essential Oils. They represent the least hazardous oils and complement each other's properties well. They each possess invaluable supporting qualities that aid meditation, relaxation, and the management of stress and stress-related conditions.

The Serenity Essential Oils

Cajeput *(Melaleuca cajuputi)*

Carrot Seed *(Daucus carota)*

Chamomile, German and Roman
(Matricaria recutita, Anthemis nobilis)

Cypress *(Cupressus sempervirens)*

Frankincense *(Boswellia carterii)*

Galbanum *(Ferula galbaniflua)*

Geranium *(Pelargonium graveolens)*

Lavender *(Lavandula angustifolia)*

Mandarin *(Citrus reticulata)*

Patchouli *(Pogostemon cablin)*

Petitgrain *(Citrus aurantium* var. *amara)*

Rose Otto *(Rosa x centifolia, R. x damascena)*

Spikenard *(Nardostachys jatamansi,
N. grandiflora)*

Tea Tree *(Melaleuca alternifolia)*

Vetivert *(Vetiveria zizanioides)*

These essential oils feature among those most frequently selected by my clients to aid their relaxation and their ability to destress, as well as to alleviate related symptoms such as insomnia, anxiety, and depression, among others. They also feature among those that appear in the historical canons, treatises, and medicinal and philosophical texts of ancient civilizations, from the ancient Chinese and Egyptians to Middle Age herbalists, alchemists, and perfumers. Knowledge about them has been recorded and passed on by shamans, priests, healers, and early doctors across time and continents.

While all Serenity Essential Oils may potentially support meditation, cypress, frankincense, galbanum, patchouli, rose otto, and spikenard have an especially pronounced influence.

ESSENTIAL OILS AND MEDITATION

Breath was, as indeed it still is, considered the portal of consciousness, the connection between the world and the Divine, the connection between the soul and the manifest material universe, the bridge between the world and the spirit within (consciousness). Breath is vital; it sustains life force. Molecules of essential oil are carried within the breath. Essential oil–impregnated breath sweeps across the olfactory bulbs as it is drawn into the nasal cavity, sending neural messages registered within the brain and detected by consciousness, and thus connecting awareness to the nuances of the internal and external world. The immediacy of odor detection, the act of deliberately smelling scent, draws the perceiver's consciousness to their breathing, to the moment.

Through the ages, fragrance has been employed to stimulate awareness of this connection, awareness of our spiritual self. Incense and resins, for example, were (and still are) burned or smoldered during rites, rituals, ceremonies, and prayer—the smoke symbolizing the soul, consciousness, rising toward heaven or the higher self. Such rites and rituals were originally performed to remind the observer to remain focused on their breath, to remain consciously connected to awareness of the omniscience of God.

Tea Tree   Citrus reticulata

Daucus carota   Ferula galbaniflua

Melaleuca alternifolia

Petitgrain Citrus aurantium **Lavender**

Nardostachys jatamansi Nardostachys grandiflora

Vetivert Pogostemon cablin **Frankincense**

Mandarin German and Roman Chamomile

Vetiveria zizanioides **Cajeput**

Lavandula angustifolia Melaleuca cajuputi

Galbanum Rosa x centifolia **Boswellia carterii**

Matricaria reticulata Anthemis nobilis

Geranium Pelargonium graveolens

Rose Otto **Carrot Seed**

Cupressus semperivirens

Patchouli

Spikenard

Cypress

Indeed, numerous references to essential oils, scented flowers, herbs, and spices are made within various scriptures including, among others, the Rig and Artharva Veda, the Quran, the Bhagavad-Gita, and the Bible. The Bible, for example, mentions several historic essences used to heal, cleanse, and protect, as well as to symbolize prayer and religious ritual. These essences, balsams, and incense were mainly extracted from crushed or infused roots, bark, twigs and leaves, or gums and resins exuding from plants and trees. (See the box on page 38.)

Essential oils can be used prior to meditation as part of your preparation process (perhaps in a bath, in a self-massage oil blend, or simply environmentally vaporized in a diffuser). They can be used during meditation to aid concentration, focus, alertness, and wakefulness, and to calm racing thoughts and ease restlessness (perhaps applied as a personal perfume or, again, diffused into the atmosphere). After meditation, essential oils can be used as a memory cue, a gentle reminder to return attention to the here and now, or for their physiological and psycho-emotional uplifting, grounding, and balancing qualities. Your

Essential Oils
(Resins, Gums, Essences, and Incense)
Referred to in the Bible

Balm of Gilead (*Pistacia lentiscus*)

Benzion styrax (*Styrax benzoin*)

Calamus (*Acorus calamus*)

Cassia (*Cinnamomum cassia*)

Cedarwood (*Cedrus atlantica*)

Cinnamon (*Cinnamomum zeylanicum*)

Frankincense (olibanum) (*Boswellia carterii*)

Galbanum (*Ferula galbaniflua*)

Labdanum (cistus, rock rose, onycha) (*Cistus ladanifer*)

Myrrh (ancient mimosa?) (*Commiphora myrrha*)

Sandalwood (possible cross-reference with aloewood, oud,
  oodh, agar) (*Santalum album*)

Spikenard (nard) (*Nardostachys jatamansi*)

References: Exodus 30:22–25, 30:34; Leviticus 2:1, 2:16, 6:16, 14:4, 14:6, 14:49, 14:51, 14:52, 24:7; Numbers 16:46–48, 19:6, 24:6; Nehemiah 8:15; Esther 2:12; Psalms 45:8, 51:7, 141:2; Proverbs 7:17, 27:9; Solomon 1:3, 1:12, 3:6, 4:6, 4:11–14, 4:13–15, 4:40; Isaiah 55:13, 60:6; Jeremiah 6:20, 8:22; Malachi 1:11; Matthew 2:11; Mark 14:3; Luke 1:10; John 19:39; Philippians 4:18; Revelations 5:8, 8:3

selection of essential oils will be personal and pertinent to you and what you require or need. There is no perfect blend in this context other than the one that works best for you at any given moment in time. Your own nose will help you discover the alchemist within; your instinct is a good starting point. The sections that follow will provide you with a lot of information that will help guide your choices.

As a very general guide to get you started, woods, tree resins, roots, and rose blossom feature among the traditional scents employed to

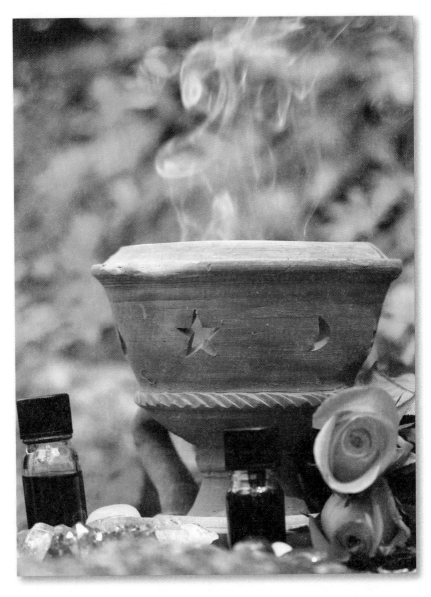

support meditation and prayer. Woods and flowers/blossoms in combination are balancing and uplifting. Woods aid breathing. Resins and roots are grounding or earthing. Spices and citrus oils are stimulating, wakening, and brightening. Herbs are balancing; some are more stimulating (rosemary, for example), some more relaxing (marjoram, for example), and some are both, such as lavender and patchouli.

HOW ARE ESSENTIAL OILS
ABSORBED BY THE BODY?

There are three ways in which essential oils may enter the body:

1. Oral ingestion (this principle also applies to rectal or vaginal absorption via suppositories or pessaries)
2. Percutaneous (skin) absorption
3. Olfactory absorption (inhalation)

Oral Ingestion

Oral ingestion **is not recommended unless prescribed and administered by a primary health-care practitioner who is also a trained and qualified essential oil practitioner; I do not advocate oral ingestion of essential oils in any other circumstance.** There are numerous cautionary factors to consider when ingesting essential oils orally. It is likely that when administered orally, 95 to 100 percent of the essential oil ingested will be absorbed into the body's internal system (unlike skin absorption, where the epidermis acts as a semiporous barrier). Essential oils should never be swallowed neat (full strength) because they can cause severe mucous membrane irritation. Although essential oils metabolize and are eliminated or excreted from the body quite quickly, there is increased risk of causing renal (kidney) and hepatic (liver) damage and internal irritation to other accessory organs of the digestive system. Some essential oils are oral toxins.

There is also increased risk of negative chemical interaction between the constituents of essential oils and other prescribed medication that may be being taken at the same time, which might potentiate or exacerbate their action. For example, sweet birch or wintergreen essential oil should never be administered internally if a person is also taking warfarin, as these essential oils dangerously increase the anticoagulant and blood-thinning potential of warfarin. In their book *Essential Oil Safety: A Guide for Health Professionals,* Tisserand and

Young particularly warn of possible incompatibility between oral ingestion of essential oils of chaste tree, cypress (blue), sandalwood (W. Australian), and jasmine sambac absolute and tricyclic antidepressants, such as imipramine and amitriptyline, or opiates, such as codeine, among other CYP2D6 substrates, because these essential oils can potentiate the action of these drugs, and other CYP1A2, CYP2C9, CYP2D6, and CYP3A4 substrates (inhalation and topical dermal application of balsam poplar, blue chamomile, sage, and yarrow may also potentiate the action of CYP2D6 substrate drugs).[3]

Percutaneous (Skin) Absorption

The skin forms part of the integumentary system and is the largest organ of the body. It provides a selective semiporous barrier that contains and protects the body's internal organs, muscles, ligaments, and bones. It regulates internal temperature through shivering or perspiration. Skin is composed of three layers: the epidermis (superficial layer), dermis (middle layer), and fatty subcutaneous tissue. The dermis contains blood and lymph vessels, nerves, and sweat and sebaceous (oil) glands that reach through the dermis to the superficial layer and hair follicles; thus the skin is both moist and oily.

Essential oils are made up of both hydrophilic (water-loving) and lipophilic (oil-loving) molecules. Because essential oils are volatile, they evaporate rapidly. Skin is generally warm to the touch, which increases the propensity for evaporation. When applied neat to the skin, hydrophilic molecules contained in essential oils bind with moisture in and on the skin; essential oil evaporation consequently instigates a drying effect and increases opportunity for irritation. Essential oils should not be applied neat to the skin. They must be appropriately diluted and suspended in vegetable oil (such as grapeseed or sweet almond), ointment, cream, or lotion. Not only do these mediums protect and moisturize the skin, they also provide lubrication, which aids application and massage and also improves absorption of essential oil molecules. (Creams and lotions, which tend to be

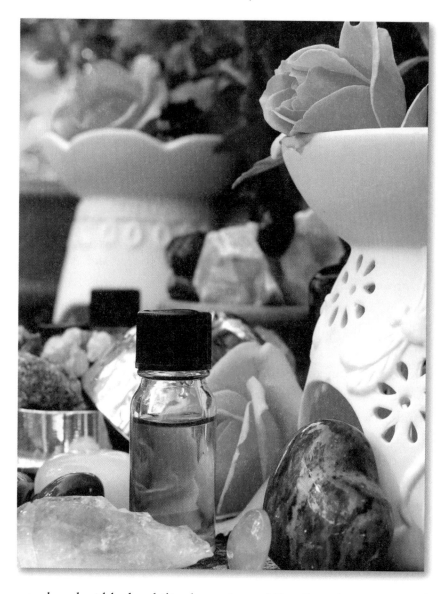

water-based, aid hydrophilic absorption, while oils and ointments aid lipophilic absorption.)

Essential oil molecules remain suspended within skin tissue for some time after application. Some of the molecules eventually filter through to capillaries, from where they are dispersed into the blood and lymphatic system and then circulate throughout the body. However, most of the essential oil will evaporate from the skin. Some molecules will be passively inhaled. Less than 10 percent of the original essential oil will actually be absorbed.[4]

Massage is a wonderful way to improve circulation (which in turn aids essential oil absorption) and aid relaxation prior to meditation. It also encourages positive feelings of self-value, respect, and compassion. Essential oils, even in minute quantities, may aid focus and concentration, ease racing thoughts, instill a sense of peace and calm, and aid breathing by clearing sinuses and encouraging deeper respiration.

Olfactory Absorption (Inhalation)

Olfaction refers to the nose and the process of the sense of smell. As a method of absorption, olfaction lends itself well to the highly volatile, odiferous nature of essential oils. As olfactory absorption relates most significantly to meditation, the entire process is covered in detail below.

Olfactory Methods of Application and Absorption

PRIMARY

Tissue or smelling strip

Steam inhalation

Perfume

Face—creams, lotions, gels, or oils

SECONDARY (EXUDING VAPORS)

Massage

Environmental diffuser

Candle-lit resin burner

Body lotions and oils

Bath oils

Shower (vaporized in steam)

Incense

OTHER SOURCES

Foods/herbs/spices

Household products

THE SENSE OF SMELL

Chemical molecules exuding from an essential oil, or from essential oils contained within and released from oil glands in flowers and plants, readily combine with oxygen molecules in the surrounding atmosphere as they evaporate. Essential oil molecules are carried with the inflow of air during breathing. Oxygen-rich air impregnated with essential oil molecules is drawn up into the nasal cavities, reaching and sweeping across the olfactory epithelium situated at the top of each cavity, before being redirected down the trachea (windpipe) into the lungs.

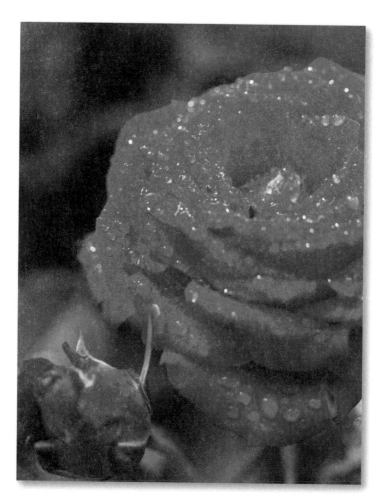

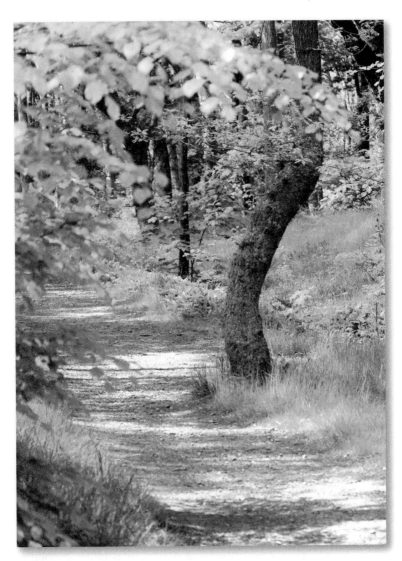

The Lungs

Passing through the nose and across the olfactory epithelium, oxygen-rich air containing essential oil molecules continues its journey down the trachea (wind pipe), into the bronchi (tubes entering the lungs), then into the lung cavity, where gaseous exchange takes place, facilitated by the alveoli (tiny specialized hollow air sacs found at the end of alveolar ducts and atria). Each lung contains around 350 million alveoli, which collectively provide approximately 80 to 120 square yards of surface area! The thin porous membrane surrounding each alveolus contains a matrix, or network, of pulmonary arterial and venal capillaries, which facilitate the movement of oxygen and carbon dioxide between air and blood.

Oxygen, along with other airborne molecules, such as those from essential oils, diffuses from the inhaled air momentarily contained within the lungs into the arterial capillaries, from where the oxygen-infused blood travels away from the lungs (through arterioles and arteries) via the circulatory system to cells throughout the body; thus essential oil molecules are carried via the blood into the internal organs and cells. The cells in exchange release carbon dioxide (CO_2) into the blood, which is carried from organs and other tissues via veins and ultimately into venal alveolar capillaries. There, along with other blood-borne volatile compounds, CO_2 diffuses out through the thin porous membrane surface into the air still held momentarily within the lungs, before being excreted from the body via exhalation of the breath.

Detection of Odorant Molecules

A certain amount of gaseous diffusion also takes place within the capillary-lined nasal cavity, pharynx, and mucous membranes en route to the lungs. Odorant molecules carried within inhaled air are deposited and dissolve in the mucous lining, which acts as a solvent, where they are detected according to their molecular shape by the correspondingly shaped cilia receptor cells (something like a key and lock). Cilia receptor cells have the capacity to provide a matrix of complex combinations (the matrix effect) that facilitate increased capacity for detection of multiple scent nuances (something like the way six lottery numbers can be combined in different sequences to form millions of potential numerical combinations).

On making contact with odorant molecules, neurons within the cilia convert (transduce) receptor activation into electrical signals, or impulses, that are relayed along the olfactory nerve to mitral cells in the olfactory bulb. Mitral cells in turn transmute the electrical impulses

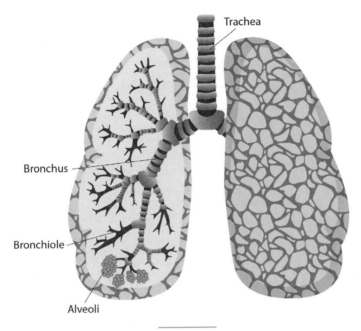

The lungs

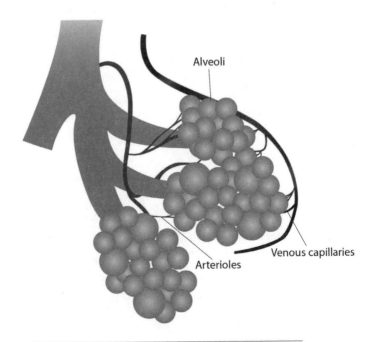

The alveoli, venous capillaries, and arterioles

they receive and relay neural signals from olfactory bulb axons along the olfactory tracts to target receptive areas within the brain that collectively form the limbic system (sometimes also referred to as the emotional brain), which includes structures such as the hypothalamus, amygdala, and hippocampus.

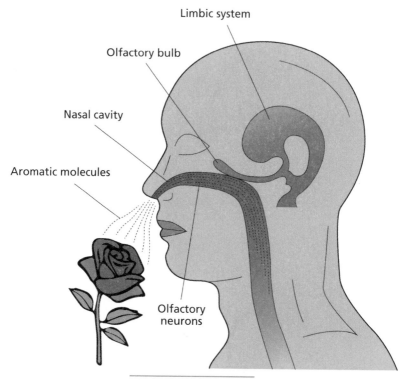

Limbic system

Olfactory bulb

Nasal cavity

Aromatic molecules

Olfactory neurons

The olfactory system

The Olfactory Journey within the Brain

Electrical signals fired from mitral cells within the olfactory bulbs travel along olfactory tract axons until these converge at the anterior commissure. This is situated centrally beneath the frontal cortex in front of the columns of the fornix at the front edge of the limbic area, central to and connecting the left and right hemispheres of the brain. The left and right nasal cavities and olfactory tracts are completely separate until reaching this point.

OLFACTION PATHWAYS INTO THE BRAIN

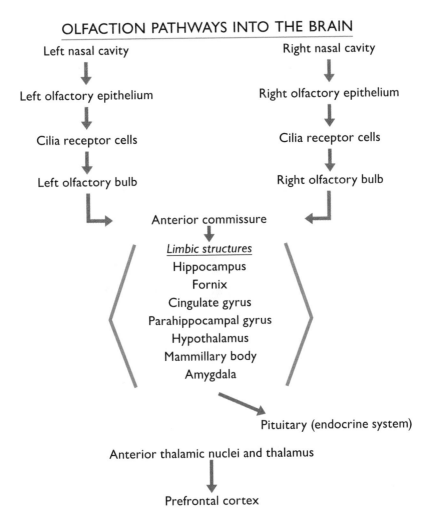

Left nasal cavity

Left olfactory epithelium

Cilia receptor cells

Left olfactory bulb

Right nasal cavity

Right olfactory epithelium

Cilia receptor cells

Right olfactory bulb

Anterior commissure

Limbic structures
Hippocampus
Fornix
Cingulate gyrus
Parahippocampal gyrus
Hypothalamus
Mammillary body
Amygdala

Pituitary (endocrine system)

Anterior thalamic nuclei and thalamus

Prefrontal cortex

The Limbic System

The limbic system comprises four major components, which form two C-shaped structures—one made up of the hippocampus and the fornix, the other made up of the cingulate gyrus and parahippocampal gyrus. The hypothalamus, mamillary body, and amygdala are also part of the limbic system. The system operates by influencing and stimulating the endocrine system and autonomic nervous system. Limbic structures associated with identifying odor, such as the amygdala and hippocampus, developed in primitive vertebrates to provide sensory signals to assist their survival (identifying food, mates, predators, dangerous chemicals exuding from rotting or noxious substances, etc.). The term *old brain* is often ascribed to areas closest to the brain stem and mid-brain where these structures are situated.

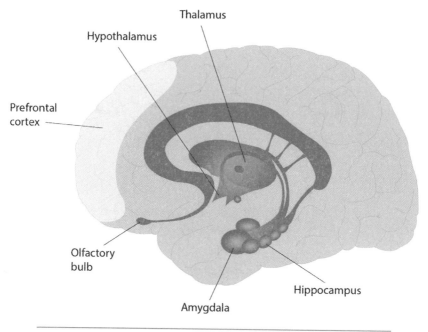

The limbic system's structure and position within the brain

Reaching from structures contained within the primitive sections of the brain to the forebrain cortex (which forms part of new mammalian brain regions), the limbic system is directly connected to the prefrontal cortex (situated in the frontal lobe) via signals relayed by dopaminergic neurotransmitters from the thalamus. Dopamine is a chemical released by nerve cells to send signals to other nerve cells found in the brain and other parts of the body. The prefrontal cortex is where the brain makes sense of, identifies, rationalizes, reasons, categorizes, and decides in relation to emotional and instinctual messages received from the limbic system (and other sensory systems such as sight, hearing, and touch).

The pituitary gland and the hypothalamus are functionally

connected to each other through attachment via the pituitary stalk. In spite of this interface, the pituitary gland (the master endocrine gland) does not form part of the limbic system. However, when we experience emotions—for example, joy or fear—these instigate the hypothalamus to influence the pituitary gland, which then releases hormones that may affect blood pressure or stimulate the heart and so on. The pituitary gland is directly involved with metabolic and physiological hormone-induced functions and processes, such as growth, regulation of blood pressure, sex organ function, thyroid gland function, water balance via the kidneys, temperature control, pain relief, and the metabolic conversion of food into energy.

How the Brain Controls Physical Movement and Function, and How It Processes Information

The human brain is separated into two *hemispheres*, the *left* and *right*; they are connected by the corpus callosum, which facilitates interhemispheric communication. Apparently the *left hemisphere* of the brain pertains to more logical thought processes and brain activity, and the *right hemisphere* to more creative ones. Physiologically, the *left hemisphere* controls neurological activity of the right side of the body, and the *right hemisphere* controls neurological activity of the left side of the body. This includes muscle control. Evidence indicates that the left hemisphere is more involved when routine or well-rehearsed processing is required and the right hemisphere is more involved in processing new situations. However, brain injury studies demonstrate that both hemispheres have equal capacity to facilitate most processes when neural pathways are redirected to undamaged parts of the brain, although there are exceptions depending on the nature and location of the damage (damage to the hippocampus, for example, can lead to irreversible long-term inability to create new memories).

DIFFERENCES BETWEEN THE
TWO HEMISPHERES OF THE BRAIN

LEFT BRAIN PROCESSING	RIGHT BRAIN PROCESSING
Analytical thought	3-D images
Components	Abstract meaning
Detail	Art awareness
Grammar	Creativity
Language	Expressiveness
Literal meaning	Face recognition
Logic	Hedonistic
Math/number skills	Holistic thought
Name recall	Imagination
Patterns	Insight
Present and past	Intuition
Rational	Music awareness
Reasoning	Philosophy and religion
Safety	Pictures
Science	Practical
Sequential control	Present and future
Theory	Risk taking
Time awareness	Spatial awareness
Words	Spontaneous
Written	Visual imagery
Masculine	Feminine
Yang	Yin

The Limbic System and Essential Oil Classification

Structures within the limbic system engage multilaterally, instantly generating a complex cluster of interactive psycho-emotional, physiological, and behavioral responses. Thus, it is very difficult to absolutely attribute, beyond general indication, specific psycho-emotional actions or to solely attribute these actions to one specific brain region, hormone, or function; there are *so many* variables at play, and they are virtually impossible to disentangle from each other.

Essential oils are, consequently, also generally therapeutically classified under umbrella terms such as *stimulating, sedating, relaxant,* and so on. However, many essential oils actually possess both stimulating and sedating properties (for example, bergamot, chamomile, clary sage, geranium, lavender, marjoram, patchouli, and ylang ylang), while others are more sedating/less stimulating or more stimulating/less sedating, rather than being purely one or the other.

Once absorbed into the body's system, essential oils appear to selectively target their action(s) to support or restore physical and psycho-emotional balance, stimulate the immune system, and act against pathogens. In their *Aromatherapy: Scent and Psyche,* aromatherapists Peter and Kate Damian point out that "essential oils . . . act to heterolaterally harmonize the brain hemispheres" and are psychoactively more quickly effective, even in small doses, when absorbed via inhalation.[5]

The box below and those on page 54 generally indicate the predominant psycho-emotional influence of essential oils, the subjective language applied to describe this influence, and the conditions essential oils may support in this context.

Primary Psycho-emotional Actions Most Commonly Cited as Being Supported by Essential Oils

Sedative/calming

Stimulant/uplifting

Balance of the central nervous system

Subjective Terms Used to Describe the Psycho-emotional Effects of Essential Oils

Balancing

Bracing

Calming

Grounding

Invigorating

Refreshing

Restorative

Strengthening

Uplifting

Warming

Psycho-emotional Conditions That Essential Oils May Ease

Anger

Anxiety

Depression

Fear

Grief

Headaches

Insomnia

Mental fog

Mental exhaustion

Mood swings

Nervous exhaustion

Nervous tension

Restlessness

Shock

Odor Receptors

Odor receptors are found in many tissues, not just the olfactory epithelium. They exist throughout the body in organ tissue (for example, liver, heart, kidneys, spleen, colon, lungs, brain, and testes) and epidermal tissue, and they are able to detect a multitude of compounds. Just as in olfactory detection, odor receptors detect molecules (lock-key) and in turn trigger and relay neural signals, which activate a cellular response. For example, odor receptors in the kidneys help control metabolic function and regulate blood pressure. Odor cells within the testes aid fertilization through attraction, guiding the sperm cell to the ovulated egg. Keratinocytes, the major cells of the epidermis, contain olfactory receptors; odor molecules stimulate these cells, affecting cell proliferation, migration, regeneration, and rejuvenation—a significant process in wound healing. Discovery of the existence of odor cells beyond the olfactory epithelium, however, is relatively recent and further research is required to identify the extent of the function of these cells. This discovery is nonetheless very significant in terms of the application of essential oils and helps explain the healing, regenerating, and rejuvenating properties, among others, of essential oils.[6]

Serenity Essential Oils and the Limbic System

All essential oils influence the limbic system in various ways, some more than others. Certain Serenity Essential Oils identified earlier in the chapter potentially have pronounced influence, as detailed below. The calming influence of frankincense, for example, aids the parasympathetic nervous system. Geranium supports a sense of emotional balance. Rose aids and supports the endocrine system, especially the reproductive system, which is regulated by the pituitary gland—as described earlier, the hypothalamus and pituitary gland (the master endocrine gland) are connected. Meditation also influences the pituitary gland to release hormones that have a calming influence on the body.

SERENITY ESSENTIAL OILS THAT POTENTIALLY HAVE A PRONOUNCED INFLUENCE ON LIMBIC SYSTEM STRUCTURES

STRUCTURE	LATIN NAME	COMMON NAME
Pituitary	*Pogostemon cablin*	Patchouli
	Rosa x damascena/centifolia	Rose
Hypothalamus	*Boswellia carterii*	Frankincense
	Pelargonium asperum/ graveolens	Geranium
Anterior thalamus	*Rosa x damascena/centifolia*	Rose
Amygdala and hippocampus	*Pelargonium asperum/ graveolens*	Geranium

Essential oils are categorized into three broad groups according to the behavior of their predominant chemical components, volatility/rate of evaporation, and fragrance profile. The term *note* is applied to these categories (in a musical sense—as in *tone, pitch, fast, slow, soft, loud, gentle, harmony,* and so on) to identify and acknowledge the multilayered, often complex qualities and nuances expressed by the various chemicals comprising an essential oil. (Consider an orchestra harmonizing the sounds of various instruments to produce a melody—each chemical within an essential oil expresses its own unique tone and each essential oil its own melody or harmony.) For ease of differentiation, each category is attributed with a color in the following table (pages 58–59): red represents *top notes* (the most volatile), blue *middle notes* (which tend to harmonize or balance the fast and slow qualities), and green *base notes* (the least volatile).

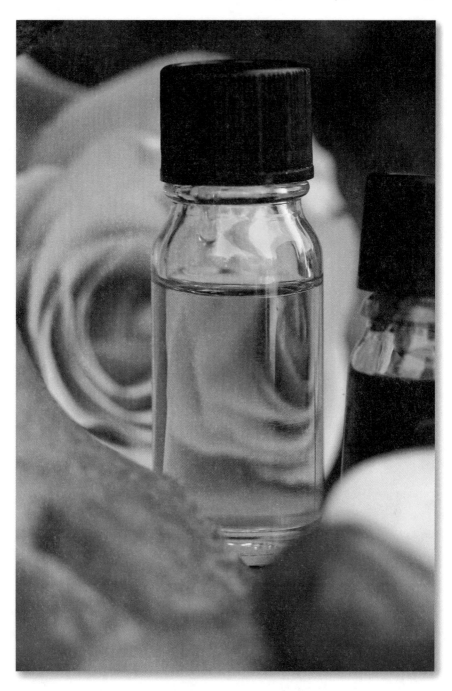

SERENITY ESSENTIAL OILS CHARACTERISTICS

	TOP NOTE	MIDDLE NOTE	BASE NOTE
TYPE OF OILS	Lemon and other citrus fruits, leaves	Herbs, flowering tops	Resins, woods, roots, blossoms
THERAPEUTIC EFFECTS	Uplifting, stimulating, revitalizing; aid memory and functions of the brain and head	Balancing, harmonizing, rejuvenating	Relaxing, earthing, sedating, calming
MAY SUPPORT / EASE (GENERAL INDICATIONS)	Extreme lethargy, melancholy, lack of interest, apathy, depression	Bodily functions, metabolism, digestion, menstruation, circulation (blood pressure)	Nervous, erratic or flighty, or hyperactive; chronic and/or long-standing conditions, the elderly; anxiety
ACTION	Fast	Moderate	Slow
SKIN PENETRATION	½ hour to 1 hour	2 hours to 3 hours	4 hours to 6 hours or more
EVAPORATION RATE	0 to 30 minutes	Up to 8 hours	Up to 12 to 24 hours, a week, sometimes longer
VOLATILITY RATE (SCALE 1 TO 100)	*Most volatile:* 1 to 14	15 to 60	*Least volatile:* 61 to 100
GENERAL FRAGRANCE CHARACTERISTIC	Sharpish	Round, soft edges	Heavy, rich, intense
EVAPORATION AND "DRY OUT" SCENT BEHAVIOR AND CHARACTERISTICS	Fresh, distinctive cluster of fragrances; obvious, light, and potentially intense due to rapid evaporation	Lingering traces of top notes; heart of the bouquet, the character; softer edges (not sharp)	Lingering traces of middle notes; faint, faded, subtle, and nondescript or heavy, tenacious residue

ESSENTIAL OILS		
Cajeput	Carrot seed	Cypress*
Galbanum	Chamomile(s)	Frankincense*
Mandarin	Cypress*	Patchouli
Petitgrain*	Frankincense*	Rose*
Tea tree	Geranium	Spikenard*
	Lavender	Vetivert
	Petitgrain*	
	Rose*	
	Spikenard*	

*The fragrance and therapeutic characteristics and behaviors of some essential oils overlap into adjacent notes, depending on their source (the part or type of plant), chemical constituents, and volatility rate. General categorization sometimes differs between authors. Those essential oils marked with an asterisk (*) sit on the border between two categories and may be placed in either one or the other.

The italics indicate the oil's secondary position (i.e., the category it may move toward). For example, petitgrain is indicated as a *top to middle* note, frankincense a *base to middle* note, and cypress a *middle to base* note.

To maintain a link between the *fast and slow elements (top and base) and to reduce rapid evaporation of more volatile components, include at least one middle note in all blends.*

The following table lists the potential psycho-emotional qualities of each Serenity Essential Oil in relation to the limbic system. As in the previous table, red indicates top notes, blue indicates middle notes, and green is used for the base notes.

THE GENERAL PSYCHO-EMOTIONAL ACTION OF SERENITY ESSENTIAL OILS AND THE POTENTIAL ASSOCIATED LIMBIC STRUCTURES INFLUENCED

ESSENTIAL OIL	POTENTIAL ASSOCIATED LIMBIC STRUCTURE	POTENTIAL CHARACTERISTIC PSYCHO-EMOTIONAL ACTION AND SUPPORT
TOP NOTES		
Cajeput (Melaleuca cajuputi)	Anterior thalamus	Aids concentration, clears and stimulates the mind, clears thoughts, helps find courage in finding new pathways and managing change, strengthens resolve and spirit
Galbanum (Ferula galbaniflua)	Hypothalamus	Balancing; both sedative and stimulant; calms erratic moods, nervous tension, menopausal symptoms, premenstrual syndrome (PMS), stress, and stress-related conditions; tonic; lifts mood and is restorative (nerves)
Mandarin (Citrus reticulata)	Hypothalamus, amygdala	Awakens; brings out the inner child; good for quelling anxiety, depression, and low mood, hyperactivity (although orange can encourage hyperactivity, mandarin is calming), insomnia, nervous tension, panic attacks, premenstrual syndrome (PMS), restlessness, stress, and stress-related conditions; has a sedative quality
Petitgrain (Citrus aurantium var. amara)	Anterior thalamus, hypothalamus	Eases anger, anxiety, depression, hyperactivity, insomnia, mental fog, nervous exhaustion, nervous tension, premenstrual syndrome (PMS), sense of hopelessness, stress, and stress-related conditions; nervous system sedative
Tea tree (Melaleuca alternifolia)	Anterior thalamus, hypothalamus	Revitalizing and stimulating; helpful for apathy, cleansing, nervous exhaustion, and shock

ESSENTIAL OIL	POTENTIAL ASSOCIATED LIMBIC STRUCTURE	POTENTIAL CHARACTERISTIC PSYCHO-EMOTIONAL ACTION AND SUPPORT
MIDDLE NOTES		
Carrot seed (Daucus carota)	Anterior thalamus, hypothalamus	Eases anxiety and apathy; calms experience of stress and confusion; helps with inability to move on, indecision, and mental and emotional exhaustion; nervous system sedative; revitalizing; aids mental clarity
Chamomile, German (Matricaria recutita)	Anterior thalamus, hypothalamus	Eases anxiety; calms experience of stress, headaches, insomnia, migraine, mood swings, nervous tension and premenstrual syndrome (PMS); mental (calms an active mind) and nervous system sedative
Chamomile, Roman Anthemis nobilis)	Anterior thalamus, hypothalamus, amygdala	Eases anger and anxiety; calms experience of stress, fear, hyperactivity, impatience, insomnia, irritability, premenstrual syndrome (PMS), restlessness, and solar plexus tension; mental, emotional, and nervous system sedative
Cypress (Cupressus sempervirens)	Anterior thalamus, hypothalamus, amygdala/ hippocampus	Eases anger, anxiety, confusion and indecision, dwelling on unpleasant events, grief and bereavement, impatience, inability to move on, irritability and intolerance, lack of concentration, nervous tension, and premenstrual syndrome (PMS); regulates autonomic nervous system, stress and stress-related conditions, and uncontrolled crying; sedative
Geranium (Pelargonium graveolens)	Anterior thalamus, hypothalamus	Both sedative and stimulant; eases anxiety, depression and low mood, headaches, jealousy, nervous tension, menopausal problems, mood swings, premenstrual syndrome (PMS), stress, and stress-related conditions; balances the nerves and solar plexus; uplifting; endocrine stimulant (hormone-like)

ESSENTIAL OIL	POTENTIAL ASSOCIATED LIMBIC STRUCTURE	POTENTIAL CHARACTERISTIC PSYCHO-EMOTIONAL ACTION AND SUPPORT
Lavender (Lavandula angustifolia)	Anterior thalamus, hypothalamus, amygdala	Sedative at low dose, stimulant at high dose; eases agitation, anger, anxiety, depression, grief and bereavement, headaches, insomnia, irritability and intolerance, manic depression (professional support required), mood swings, nervous tension, panic, premenstrual syndrome (PMS), sense of hopelessness, shock, solar plexus tension, stress and stress-related conditions, suspicion
BASE NOTES		
Frankincense (Boswellia carterii)	Anterior thalamus, hypothalamus, amygdala/ hippocampus	Eases anger, anxiety, confusion and indecision, depression and low mood, dwelling on unpleasant events, fear and paranoia, grief and bereavement, hyperactivity, impatience, inability to move on, irritability and intolerance, mood swings, nervous tension, panic attacks (calms and relaxes breathing), premenstrual syndrome (PMS), resentment and disappointment, sadness and despair; sedative; helps let go of unwanted thoughts and memories; supports meditation and finding inner tranquility
Patchouli (Pogostemon cablin)	Anterior thalamus, hypothalamus	Sedative at low dose, stimulant at high dose; eases apathy, confusion and indecision, depression and low mood, nervous exhaustion, nervous tension, panic attacks, premenstrual syndrome (PMS), and stress and stress-related conditions; endocrine stimulant; supports meditation and a sense of spirituality
Rose Otto (Rosa x damascena, Rosa x centifolia)	Anterior thalamus, hypothalamus, amygdala	Sedative at low dose, stimulant at high dose; eases agitation, anger, anxiety, depression (especially postnatal) and low mood, fear and paranoia, grief and bereavement (and sense of loss), hatred, headaches (tension and hormonal), hypersensitivity, insomnia, jealousy, migraine, nervous tension, panic attacks, premenstrual syndrome (PMS), resentment and disappointment, sadness and despair, and stress and stress-related conditions; endocrine stimulant (hormone-like); aphrodisiac

ESSENTIAL OIL	POTENTIAL ASSOCIATED LIMBIC STRUCTURE	POTENTIAL CHARACTERISTIC PSYCHO-EMOTIONAL ACTION AND SUPPORT
Spikenard (*Nardostachys jatamansi, Nardostachys grandiflora*)	Anterior thalamus, hypothalamus	Balances sympathetic nervous system with parasympathetic nervous system (tonic to the sympathetic nervous system, regulates the parasympathetic nervous system); grounding; eases anxiety, grief and bereavement, hatred, headaches and migraine, hyperactivity, hysteria, impatience, insomnia, intolerance, irritability, menopausal symptoms, nervous indigestion, nervous tension, panic attacks, PMS, restlessness, and stress and stress-related conditions; sedative
Vetivert (*Vetiveria zizanioides*)	Anterior thalamus, hypothalamus, amygdala	Reduces symptoms of withdrawal when coming off medication (especially tranquilizers); balances the central nervous system, eases anxiety, confusion and indecision, debility, depression, hyperactivity, hypersensitivity, impatience, insomnia, mental exhaustion, menopausal symptoms, nervous tension, panic attacks, premenstrual syndrome, and stress and stress-related conditions; sedative (especially for the nervous system), earthing, and grounding

The diagram on page 64 provides an "at a glance" overview of Serenity Essential Oils' multidynamic qualities. This guide, or map, places the oils into functional categories based on their predominant actions—from physiological to psycho-emotional to their ambient aesthetic and hedonistic perfume qualities—which will aid you in quickly and easily selecting an appropriate essential oil for a given requirement.

WHAT SERENITY ESSENTIAL OILS OFFER
(topical non-oral and environmental use only)

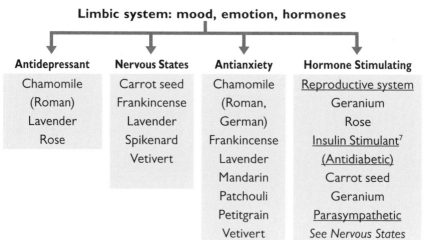

PSYCHOLOGICAL
Limbic system: mood, emotion, hormones

Antidepressant	Nervous States	Antianxiety	Hormone Stimulating
Chamomile (Roman)	Carrot seed	Chamomile (Roman, German)	Reproductive system
Lavender	Frankincense	Frankincense	Geranium
Rose	Lavender	Lavender	Rose
	Spikenard	Mandarin	Insulin Stimulant[7] (Antidiabetic)
	Vetivert	Patchouli	Carrot seed
		Petitgrain	Geranium
		Vetivert	Parasympathetic *See Nervous States*

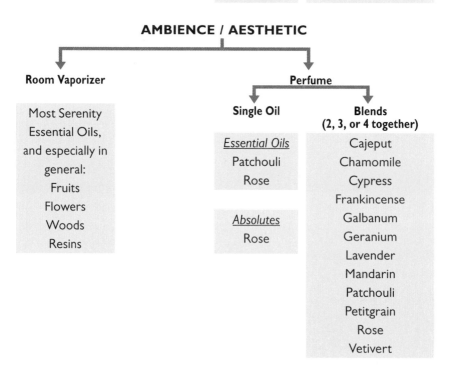

AMBIENCE / AESTHETIC

Room Vaporizer

Perfume

	Single Oil	Blends (2, 3, or 4 together)
Most Serenity Essential Oils, and especially in general:	*Essential Oils* Patchouli Rose	Cajeput Chamomile Cypress Frankincense
Fruits Flowers Woods Resins	*Absolutes* Rose	Galbanum Geranium Lavender Mandarin Patchouli Petitgrain Rose Vetivert

EXPLORING THE PSYCHO-EMOTIONAL AND PHYSIOLOGICAL EFFECTS OF ESSENTIAL OILS

The brain is responsive to external sensory input and neurological stimulation and facilitates internal homeostasis, environmental awareness, consciousness of a deeper sense of being, and relationships with other people and the external world. Fragrance detection triggers numerous neurological, physiological, emotional, and hedonistic responses at the same time, which are difficult to disentangle. While it may be very difficult to prove or explain specifically *how* essential oils affect the brain, their vaporizing odorous molecules do instigate (to varying degrees) neurological responses that appear to affect mood, emotion, memory, concentration, and cognition (either via inhalation or circulatory absorption), even if this influence is only temporary. Meanwhile, research and deliberation continue in a quest for better understanding.

Indeed, there are numerous studies (mainly conducted by or on behalf of the food and manufacturing, cosmetic, and pharmaceutical industries) exploring the psychotherapeutic effects of essential oils on attention, concentration, productivity, mental-emotional stimulation and sedation, mood states (anxiety, depression, agitation, restlessness), memory, and insomnia. Several studies are described here, along with their conclusions to date.

Studies using animals, such as mice, although ethically controversial, eliminate many potentially influential *subjective* psycho-emotional variables when exploring the basic physiological and behavioral effects of essential oils and provide very useful indications. However, these studies do not completely reflect the real complexities of true-life scenarios when applied to humans, where the idiosyncratic psycho-emotional and hedonistic responses to essential oils contribute to the outcome of their actions, or, conversely, the complex influence essential oils actually have on the individual's psyche, cognition, and physiological function (the inside-out, outside-in response).

In their 1993 study "Fragrance Compounds and Essential Oils with Sedative Effects upon Inhalation," testing the ability of essential oils to calm motility (spontaneous movement) in mice, Buchbauer and associates confirmed the sedative effects of lavender, neroli (orange blossom), linalool and linalyl acetate (isolated chemical components), and citronella when inhaled at low concentration (blood samples revealed the absorption of fragrance compounds), and they concluded that "the results contribute to the correct interpretation of the term 'aromatherapy' (i.e. a stimulating or sedative effect on the behavior of individuals upon inhalation of fragrance compounds)."[8] A similar study conducted by Kovar et al. in 1987 demonstrated the sedative effect of rosemary essential oil on the locomotor activity of mice after inhalation, which they attributed in particular to 1,8-cineole, a component of rosemary detected in blood samples post-exposure.[9]

In another study involving 144 human subjects in 2003, Mark Moss, head of Northumbria University's psychology department, and associates compared the effects of essential oils of rosemary and lavender on cognition and mood in one subject group and no essential oil in the control group, to test memory and mental alertness. The participants were aware of the task they were performing, but were not aware that essential oils formed part of the study. The essential oils were diffused into the environment while recipients were engaged in various cognitive tasks. They found that essential oils of lavender (*Lavandula angustifolia*) and rosemary (*Rosmarinus officinalis*) significantly affected aspects of cognitive performance. Lavender decreased the performance of working memory, impairing alertness and retention time for both memory and attention-based tasks, while rosemary improved the quality and speed of working memory and secondary memory and increased alertness; both lavender and rosemary reportedly also produced feelings of contentment during tasks.[10] In a subsequent smaller study in 2012, Moss and Oliver reiterated this finding when testing for speed, accuracy, and evaluation of mood during mathematical tasks where twenty-two subjects were exposed to rosemary essential oil, observing correlation between the higher levels of 1,8-cineole and improved performance.[11]

However, Ilmberger and associates' study "The Influence of Essential Oils on Human Attention" found no significant difference in terms of core attentional function in the presence of essential oils but did observe complex correlation between subjective evaluation of substances and objective task performance. This consequently led to their suggestion that the effects of essential oils (in this case, peppermint, jasmine, and ylang ylang) or their components (1,8-cineole, menthol) on basic forms of attentional behavior are actually mainly *psychological,* and that a subject's *expectation* of an odor may affect motivation and subsequent behavior.[12]

In his 2001 paper "Attention Deficit and Hyperactivity Disorder (ADHD)," Terry S. Friedmann, M.D., examined the effectiveness of essential oils of lavender (*Lavandula angustifolia*), cedarwood (*Cedrus atlantica*), and vetivert (*Vetiveria zizanioides*), which were applied to improve the focus and attention of children aged between six and fourteen years diagnosed as presenting with ADHD (attention deficit hyperactive disorder). EEG (electro-encephalograph) equipment was used to measure beta and theta brain wave activity in areas of the brain before and after a thirty-day period of exposure to one of the three essential oils subjects were asked to inhale, holding the open bottle next to the nostrils and taking three deep breaths, three times per day; the placebo group received no treatment. The results demonstrated significant improvement in brain activity and reduction of symptoms of ADHD for vetivert (100%), slightly less for cedarwood (83%), and no apparent improvement for lavender (53%), supporting Moss et al.'s 2003 experimental finding.[13]

In their 2002 study "Aromatherapy as a Safe and Effective Treatment for the Management of Agitation in Severe Dementia," King's College London professor Clive G. Ballard et al. found that melissa (lemon balm) essential oil, when added to a base lotion and applied twice a day to the arms and faces of seventy-two elderly subjects with severe dementia, significantly relieved their agitation; the placebo group received the same treatment, using sunflower oil in place of the melissa (lemon balm) in the lotion. Although this treatment was applied in a topical lotion to the skin, subjects were also exposed to inhalation of the melissa because the lotion was applied to the face, and therefore under their nose.[14]

Elaine Perry, professor of neurochemical pathology at Newcastle University, in a review examining the effectiveness of aromatherapy for the treatment of dementia, reported in 2014 that application of lavender and lemon balm (melissa) increased functional abilities and communication and decreased difficult behavior. Perry also reported that a blend of lavender, marjoram, patchouli, and vetivert applied in a cream to the skin of elderly patients (again, considering the effects of inhalation) increased their alertness, contentment, and ability to sleep at night and reduced levels of agitation, withdrawal, and wandering.[15]

In a 2012 study, "Short-Term Study on the Effects of Rosemary on Cognitive Function in an Elderly Population," Andrew Pengelly et al. found that rosemary (in dried, powdered form), when consumed orally in low dose (750 mg), similar to its usual culinary consumption, improved the speed of memory in twenty-eight elderly subjects (average age seventy-five years), but that at high dose (6,000 mg) it significantly impaired memory function (thus highlighting also that the dose, or quantity, is significant for the whole herb, but especially for essential oils, which consists of concentration of the plant's volatile components; only very small amounts of essential oil are necessary to procure odor detection and a potential cephalic response).[16]

Speed of memory is used as an indicator of cognitive function in the elderly when testing for Alzheimer's disease or dementia. In a study published in *Psychogeriatrics* in 2009, Jimbo et al. found that a blend of rosemary essential oil with lemon essential oil and a blend of lavender essential oil with orange essential oil improved personal orientation related to cognitive function in elderly patients diagnosed with Alzheimer's disease or dementia. They concluded that aromatherapy is an efficacious nonpharmacological therapy with some potential for improving cognitive function, especially for those with Alzheimer's.[17]

In 2002 Haze et al. reported in the *Japanese Journal of Pharmacology* on their investigation of the effects of inhalation of essential oils on sympathetic nervous system activity in normal adult subjects, measuring blood pressure and plasma catecholamine levels from blood samples. Results showed that "inhalation of essential oils, such as black pepper oil, estragon oil, fennel oil or grapefruit oil, resulted in a 1.5 to 2.5-fold *increase* in relative sympathetic activity, compared with inhalation of an odorless solvent (triethyl citrate)" and, "in contrast, fragrant inhalation of rose oil or patchouli oil caused a 40% *decrease* in relative sympathetic activity," concluding that "fragrance inhalation of essential oils may modulate sympathetic activity in normal adults."[18] Chang and Chen (2011) investigated the effect of bergamot essential oil on the autonomic nervous system, and more specifically as an antidote to the psycho-physiological consequence of stress experienced in the workplace. Subjects were exposed to the essential oil, which was dispensed in an essential oil ionizer diffuser or spray, for ten minutes. Blood pressure and heart rate were measured before, during, and after exposure to the essential oil. Results indicated that essential oils appear to "drive autonomic nervous activity toward a balanced state."[19]

In a 1999 article "Odours and Mental States," J. Stephan Jellinek suggests that the pharmacological mechanism is far less dominant when it comes to affecting psychological states and that psychodynamic odor effects, although difficult to prove conclusively, may be based on:

a) A quasi-*pharmacological* mechanism influencing the central nervous system or hormonal systems.

b) A *semantic* mechanism accounting for the influence of personal experiences with certain odors.

c) A *hedonic* valence mechanism providing the dimension for pleasantness for emotional states.

d) A *placebo* mechanism, which is based on subjective expectation.[20]

The following table, adapted from Jellinek, illustrates his findings.

COMPARING PHARMACOLOGICAL AND PSYCHODYNAMIC ODOR EFFECTS

INFLUENCING FACTOR	PHARMACOLOGICAL	SEMANTIC	HEDONISTIC	PLACEBO
Biological	☺		☺	
Personal Experience		☺	☺	☺
Cultural Experience		☺	☺	☺
Personality				☺
Olfactory Acuity		☺	☺	
Stimulus Characteristic	Chemical	Odor	Odor	Reputation

In a more recent (2013) double-blind, placebo-controlled clinical study evaluating the effect of aromatherapy with *Rosa damascena* on the perception of post-surgery pain in children aged three to six years, Maryam Marofi et al. observed significant reduction in pain after diffusion of the rose. Sixty-four children (with the consent of their parent or guardian, and ethical clearance from the hospital's clinical research department) were randomly divided into two groups (A and B). The children in group A were given the essential oil (rose) and the children in group B were given only a carrier oil, sweet almond. Both groups otherwise received exactly the same prescribed post-surgical care. A postoperative pain assessment (TPPPS—Toddler Preschooler Postoperative Pain Scale) was carried out as soon as the children were submitted to their ward. Then an eye pad infused with one or two drops of either rose essential oil or sweet almond oil was placed 12 inches from the child's head. The pain assessment was repeated at 3, 6, 9, and 12 hours after surgery. Although there was initially little difference between both groups after the first assessment, and although there was some reduction of post-operative pain in both groups over the test period, the subsequent assessments did reveal significant decrease in the average score of pain intensity for the essential oil group. These children were probably too young to have formulated subjective or sematic expectation of the scent. The pleasant sweetness of the scent may have stimulated a hedonistic/placebo response. However, the odor molecules may also have stimulated an independent biological/pharmacological reaction too.[21]

MEMORY

Odor memory is more tenacious compared with other senses (sight, sound, touch, hearing). Memory is reinforced and enhanced and may last or linger longer where multiple sensory stimulations occur at the same time. This is especially so when less consciously controlled cognitive processes, which do not involve judgment, deliberation, reasoning, or rational evaluation, are being performed, such as creative tasks, learning or performing by rote, and so on (this works the same for negative and positive experiences). Thus, activities such as massage, meditation, visualization, or relaxation techniques may be positively enhanced and experientially memorably reinforced when complementary essential oils are vaporized at the same time (and vice versa).

Rachel Herz, assistant professor in the department of psychiatry and human behavior at Brown University, is an expert on the psychological science of smell. While exploring the role of odor-evoked memories, she significantly observed that any scent that evokes a happy autobiographical memory for a given individual has the potential to increase positive emotions, decrease negative moods, lower stress, and decrease inflammatory immune responses. She also found that odor-evoked memories may stimulate specific emotions, such as self-confidence, motivation, and vigor. Herz found that memories elicited by odors are more emotionally potent than memories evoked by other sensory stimuli, and when salient emotion is experienced during odor exposure, the effectiveness of an odor memory cue is enhanced, illustrated through observed increase in activity in the amygdala.[22]

In a 2000 study "Aromatherapy and Children with Learning Difficulties," Vicky Pitman exploited this salient connection between scent and memory to help hyperactive children manage their restlessness, using visualization and self-massage during exposure to selected essential oils to instill a sense of calmness and peace that could be recalled and experienced later when deliberately inhaling the scent of the same essential oil(s) as a memory cue, applied and used to calm their behavior and assist their focus on tasks. Pitman observed that "it was very noticeable that both the oils and the relaxation improved concentration. Students definitely stayed calmer longer and recovered quickly from upsets. There were fewer disruptions to lessons."[23]

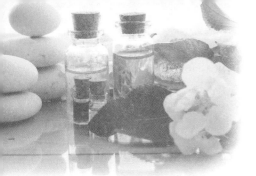

3

Applying Essential Oils

*Safety Guidelines and
Indications for Eight Therapeutic
Application Methods*

There are various methods of applying essential oils. When applied appropriately, essential oils pose little risk. However, while their therapeutic qualities are undoubtedly highly beneficial, they are best used in limited, controlled amounts, especially when applying them on a frequent or daily basis. As a general rule, six drops of essential oil per day is the appropriate, safe limit for epidermal applications (via perfume, massage, cream, lotion, ointment) or direct olfactory absorption (steam inhalation or smelling strip). I have observed through my therapeutic practice that, even when applied in very small amounts, essential oils can procure a very effective response.

The following information applies to the use of essential oils as companions for mindfulness and meditation in general.

SAFE APPLICATION GUIDELINES

I do not advocate the internal use of essential oils, unless prescribed by a professional practitioner with biomedical, pharmaceutical, or herbalist training. Awareness of the chemical interactions and physiological effects of essential oils is imperative. Essential oils are highly concentrated, volatile, odiferous chemicals, with the propensity to cause irritation and sensitization and, for some people, although relatively rare, allergic reaction, if not applied appropriately (or if stored incorrectly).

Purchasing Essential Oil

First, ensure that you purchase essential oils from a reputable supplier whose oils are fresh, correctly packaged, and appropriately labeled, and who can vouch for the integrity of the oils they supply (details of the source, location of growth, botanical family, Latin name, batch number, safety data information, and so on). Oils that are much cheaper than average are potentially not genuine and are often adulterated or bulked out with inferior, less expensive chemicals (equally, very expensive essential oils are often adulterated with cheaper substitute chemicals or essential oils to increase profit margins). Read the labels carefully to ensure that bottles or products contain 100 percent pure essential oils.

Also, only purchase essential oils stored in amber or blue glass bottles (to protect against UV light damage) with a dropper cap (this ensures careful measurement, inhibits rapid oxidization, prevents spillage, and limits accidental ingestion by children; ask for childproof lids if necessary). Never purchase or use essential oils that have been stored in plastic bottles and do not purchase essential oils that have been stored on brightly lit, warm shelves. Essential oils are highly flammable and should be kept away from fire (candles etc.) and sources of intense heat.

Second, before use, ensure that you know about the chemical and therapeutic properties of and applicable contraindications and cautions in relation to the essential oil(s) you intend to apply.

Patch Testing

Patch testing is a precautionary measure to ensure the safe application of an essential oil or blend of essential oils. It is not necessary and would be impractical to carry out a patch test every time an essential oil was considered for use. However, there are indicators that can guide this choice. For example, *a patch test is advisable* where there is:

+ A history of sensitivity or allergy to perfumes, skin-care or household products, metals or chemicals, and so on.
+ A preexisting condition such as eczema, asthma, dermatitis, or hay fever.
+ Sensitivity or allergy to a particular plant, as it is likely that the essential oil from that plant will trigger a similar event.
+ Sensitivity or allergy to particular foods or processed food additives (e.g., nuts, seeds, citrus fruits, herbs, artificial flavoring, coloring, or preservatives).
+ Current or recent long-term chronic illness (weakened immune system).

If any of these indications are present, a patch test should be conducted, following these guidelines:

+ 1 to 2 drops of essential oil, or blend of essential oils, should be diluted in the chosen carrier medium (vegetable oil, such as grapeseed or olive oil, or other carrier medium that you intend to use to apply the essential oil, such as unscented cream or lotion—as a precaution, avoid using nut oils such as almond, walnut, and hazelnut for this preliminary test).
+ Wash and dry the area of skin selected for the patch test (for example, the fold of the arm at the elbow, the wrist, or the upper forearm).
+ Apply the diluted essential oil(s) to the test area using a biodegradable cotton bud or swab.
+ Occlude (cover) the test area with a non-allergenic bandage.
+ Leave for 24 to 48 hours.
+ Avoid contact with water for the duration of the test.

✦ Remove the bandage and observe the test area for sign of irritation, guided by the International Contact Dermatitis Research Group (ICDRG) patch test scale given below.

✦ If there is no reaction, or only mild redness (the bandage can cause mild redness, which should clear once the bandage is removed), continue to use the mixture as intended.

✦ If the test outcome is positive (3 to 5 on the ICDRG scale), do not use that essential oil. Or retest each essential oil separately if a blended mixture was applied to identify which one was the antagonist; then adjust the blend accordingly.

International Contact Dermatitis Research Group (ICDRG) Patch Test Scale

1. No reaction.
2. Doubtful reaction: mild redness.
3. Weak positive reaction: red and slightly thickened skin.
4. Strong positive reaction: red swollen skin with individual small watery blisters.
5. Extreme positive reaction: intense redness and swelling with coalesced large blisters or spreading reaction (extending beyond the area of application).
6. Irritant reaction: red skin improves once patch is removed.

For more information, visit www.icdrg.org.

Essential Oils—Cautions to Observe

1. Do not swallow or take essential oils internally.
2. Do not apply essential oils neat (full strength) on the skin (always dilute in a vegetable oil or other carrier medium such as unscented cream, lotion, or ointment). Undiluted dermal application of essential oils can lead to irritation

and sensitization. Lavender and tea tree essential oils are exceptions to this rule, and they are often used as first aid remedies for insect stings, minor burns or skin abrasions, or mild skin infections. Still, repeated long-term topical application of these oils is not advisable due to the risk of sensitization (in which repeated application results in the progressive amplification of a response).

3. Keep out of the reach of children (suppliers will provide childproof lids if requested) and away from pets.

4. Accidental ingestion: *Do not induce vomiting.* Drink full-fat milk. Seek medical advice immediately. Keep the bottle the essential oil was stored in for identification (the label should have Latin name, batch number, sell-by date, etc.; the bottle will have traces of the oil).

5. Eyes: Essential oils can be transferred from fingers to the eyes (always wash your hands after using or handling essential oils). If *neat* essential oil enters your eyes, *immediately* flush with vegetable oil or full-fat milk, then rinse thoroughly with clean warm water. Sometimes diluted essential oils enter the eyes during steam inhalation, bathing, or showering; if this happens, immediately flush eyes with clean warm water. In either case, seek medical advice *immediately* if irritation or stinging persists after flushing the eye(s).

6. Skin reaction: Apply vegetable oil to dilute the essential oil on the skin, then thoroughly wash the area with non-perfumed soap (liquid soap if possible) and rinse with warm water to remove any trace of soap and the essential oil. Dry the area thoroughly and apply an unscented base cream (vegetable oil or even butter if nothing else is available) to soothe irritation if appropriate.

7. Only purchase essential oils from reputable suppliers (who will provide safety data information).

8. Only purchase essential oils stored in amber or dark blue glass bottles with dropper-top lids (to ensure careful measurement and prevent spillage or accidental ingestion).

9. Check the sell-by date before use and make a note of the date of purchase. Essential oils oxidize rapidly when exposed to oxygen in the atmosphere. They therefore have a limited shelf life: 2 years if unopened, 1 year once opened (citrus oils, such as mandarin, have a shelf life of just 6 months once opened).

10. Never "top up" a bottle of essential oil with more essential oil once opened for use.

11. Discard small amounts of essential oil left in a bottle or container, unless you have been rapidly using up the essential oil from the moment of first opening the bottle.

12. Replace lids immediately after use (to slow down oxidization).

13. Store in a cool dark place, away from sources of heat and direct sunlight (preferably a fridge—although some oils, such as rose otto, will solidify when very cold, they will return to a liquid state at room temperature).

14. Wipe up spillages immediately (essential oils will dissolve/damage polystyrene, plastic, varnish, paint, and polished and laminated surfaces).

Measuring Essential Oils

It is very important to measure essential oils carefully, as they are prone to cause skin and mucous membrane irritation and sensitivity if over-used or inappropriately applied. Measurement percentages can seem quite complicated, especially considering that dropper-top sizes vary, rendering absolute accuracy impossible. However, in the interest of safety, essential oil quantities do need to be monitored. Therefore, as a "rule of thumb guide," assume the averages set out in the measurement guide on page 79.

Risk of sensitivity or irritation reactions increases where large amounts of essential oil are applied to very small areas of skin—applying six drops of essential oil in a carrier medium to the whole body through massage will have negligible irritant effect, yet the same quantity of essential oil applied to a small area of skin can be irritant, particularly in sensitive areas such as the face, underarms, and so on.

Use no more than one or two drops of essential oils in a carrier medium on localized areas of skin. Keep this in mind when making first aid ointments or face creams or lotions. When making face creams and so on for regular use, reduce the amount of essential oils included, change the essential oil selection from time to time, and have "no essential oil" breaks occasionally.

Measurement Guide

5 ml (approximately 0.17 fl oz) = 100 drops of essential oil

10 ml (approximately 0.34 fl oz) = 200 drops of essential oil

---

The maximum amount of essential oil per twenty-four-hour period for a healthy adult is six to ten drops. Apply for two to three weeks only, followed by one week's abstinence, and change the essential oil(s) selection regularly.

The following guide will help you work out the percentage of a blend of essential oils and a carrier medium such as vegetable oil, cream, lotion, ointment, or gel.

Proportions of Essential Oil and Carrier Medium = Blend Percentage

1 drop of essential oil in 5 ml of carrier medium = 1% blend

2½ drops of essential oil in 5 ml of carrier medium = 2.5% blend (round up or down)

5 drops of essential oil in 5 ml of carrier medium = 5% blend

---

Appropriate Quantities

The appropriate quantities of essential oils are indicated by the age and robustness or frailty of the individual, along with other factors such as allergies or asthma. The following are the recommended number of drops and resulting blend percentages for normal adult use and for both reduced and exceptional amounts.

Reduced Amounts

I personally do not advocate direct application of essential oils for infants under twelve months, even in dilution; internal organs are not fully matured until after this period. The following information is included in the interest of safety. Do not directly apply essential oils, in any circumstances, to infants between birth and three months old. For infants between three months and twenty-four months old, use the **maximum dilution—that is, 1 drop of essential oil in 20 ml or more of carrier medium—**and **do not use herbaceous, spicy, or citrus oil.**

The following amounts are appropriate for children, for those who are frail or very elderly, and for those with sensitivities, allergies, eczema, or asthma, as well as for facial blends.

(a) 1 drop of essential oil in 5 ml of carrier medium = 1% blend
     2 drops of essential oil in 10 ml of carrier medium = 1% blend

(b) 1 drop of essential oil in 10 ml of carrier medium = 0.5% blend
     2 drops of essential oil in 20 ml of carrier medium = 0.5% blend

(c) 1 drop of essential oil in 20 ml of carrier medium = 0.25% blend

Normal Amount

For general and adult use:

2½ drops of essential oil in 5 ml of carrier medium = 2.5% blend
(round up or down)
5 drops of essential oil in 10 ml of carrier medium = 2.5% blend

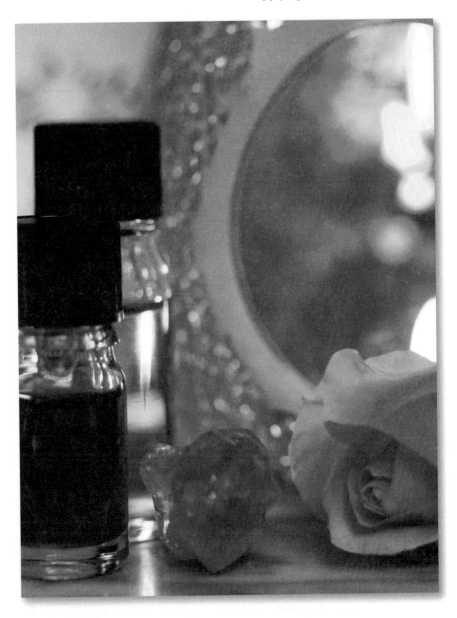

Acute / Exceptional Amount

For acute, short-term occasional use. Avoid or reduce the use of known irritant oils.

5 drops of essential oil in 5 ml of carrier medium = 5% blend
10 drops of essential oil in 10 ml carrier medium = 5% blend

The following general application guidelines are relevant to essential oil use for all eight of the methods presented in this chapter.

Applying Essential Oils:
General Guidelines

1. Decide on your specific purpose or theme to hone your essential oil selection, whether it is to aid relaxation, to stimulate alertness, to create a particular ambience, to aid a particular emotion (uplifting, grounding, balancing), to aid meditation, and so on.

2. It's OK to use a single, specially selected essential oil; however, a pertinent well-chosen essential oil can be equally effective as a blend of two or three essential oils.

3. If you decide to use more than one essential oil in a blend, limit them to three or four essential oils and affirm their compatibility, or harmony, with each other.

4. When using more than one essential oil, aim to include different notes to enhance the balance and tenacity of your blend (remember, base note essential oils linger longest, and top notes evaporate very quickly).

5. Avoid blending stimulating essential oils with relaxing essential oils.

6. Avoid using the same essential oil or blend of essential oils repeatedly. Change your selection from time to time. If you are using essential oils regularly for their psycho-emotional qualities, apply reduced amounts; less is more when applying over long periods of time.

7. Take periods of abstinence. For example, use your essential oils for three or four weeks and then have a week's break. Changing the essential oil or the blended combinations you use will aid in avoiding sensitization to a particular essential oil or chemical component(s) found within the oil(s).

8. Stop using your selected essential oil or essential oil blend immediately if you feel nauseous or develop a headache or skin rash, redness, or itchiness (particularly at the point of application).

9. If vaporizing essential oils in a communal or public area, ensure those people sharing the area agree/are aware that you are vaporizing essential oils. Do not take it for granted that everyone likes the scent of essential oils or those *you* like and select.

ROLLER BOTTLES

Roller bottles are best used for the application of therapeutic and aesthetic perfumes. They are convenient, safe, and easy to use.

Method
Half fill a a 10-ml roller bottle with a carrier oil, such as jojoba, borage seed, grapeseed, and so on (do not use mineral oil). Add up to 10 drops of your chosen essential oil or blend of essential oils. Top up with carrier oil to the shoulder of the bottle. Secure the roller ball cap and lid. Roll the bottle rapidly between the palms and fingers of your hands to shake up and disperse the essential oils throughout the carrier oil. Leave in a cool place to stand for 24 hours to allow essential oils to diffuse evenly into the carrier oil.

Remove the external cap and roll the perfume oil onto your wrists or temples as and when required, replacing the lid immediately after use (use within 6 weeks).

NB: For personal application only. The roller bottle can be reused (and/or recycled)—wash with warm soapy water, rinse, and dry thoroughly before refilling (or recycling).

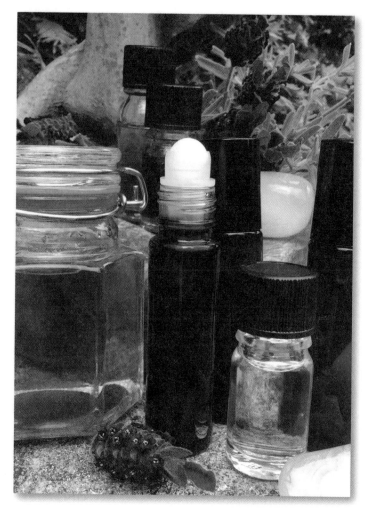

Indications

Use for:

+ Aesthetic purposes—attractant, mood, occasion, theme
+ Anxiety and depression
+ Headaches
+ Improving or reinforcing memory retention
+ Psycho-emotional moods and conditions—for example, for grief, joy, loss, nervousness, or pleasure; or to balance, calm, invigorate, sedate, or uplift
+ Stress-related conditions

NASAL INHALERS

Nasal inhalers are for therapeutic use. They are convenient and safe, even for older children, as there is no direct contact with the essential oil(s). Designed for direct personal inhalation, they are more discreet than other applications such as a perfume. Nasal inhalers offer a clean and efficient way of inhaling essential oils with immediate effect on the respiratory system (throat and lungs) and limbic system (mood, emotions, and mental clarity). They can be carried around in a pocket or bag and applied as and when required.

Method

Dismantle the nasal inhaler to remove the wadding roll inside the containing tube. Add 2 to 6 drops of your selected essential oil or blend of essential oils to the wadding roll. Replace the essential oil–infused wadding into the containing tube, secure the small base cap to seal the wadding within the

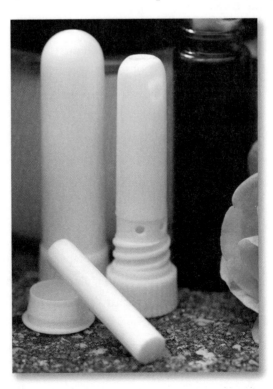

tube, then screw on the protective cover. Remove the cover, then holding the tube to your nose, inhale through each nostril as required. Replace the protective cover immediately after use to contain the essential oil vapors.

NB: For personal application only. The plastic container can be reused (and/or recycled)—wash with warm soapy water, rinse, and dry thoroughly before reusing (or recycling). Replace the wadding roll with a roll of cotton wool or tissue. Do not reuse more than two or three times.

Indications

Use for:

+ Anxiety and depression
+ Chest infections
+ Colds and flu
+ Headaches
+ Immune support (antimicrobial, anti-infectious, antiviral)
+ Improving or reinforcing memory retention
+ Improving respiration
+ Insomnia
+ Mental clarity (to clear head and thoughts)
+ Psycho-emotional moods and conditions—for example, for grief, joy, loss, nervousness, or pleasure, or to balance, calm, invigorate, or uplift
+ Sinus congestion
+ Sore throat
+ Stress and stress-related conditions

TISSUES

Tissues are a quick and easy method of therapeutic inhalation. When you add a couple drops of essential oil to a clean tissue, the essential oil molecules are able vaporize freely with full and immediate impact and benefit. (Vaporization is limited when smelling an essential oil directly from the bottle.) This method offers a useful first aid remedy for headaches, shock and upset, and colds and flu.

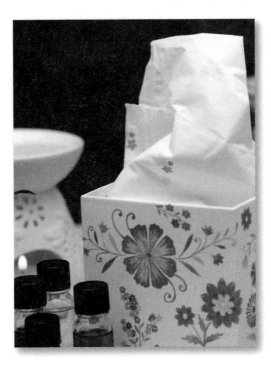

Method

Add 1 to 3 drops of your selected essential oil or blend of essential oils to the tissue. Inhale the vapors from the tissue as required. Do not allow essential oil–infused tissue to touch the skin on your face or nose to avoid potential skin irritation.

For Immediate Need or First Aid

Here is a useful method for cases of immediate need or for first aid, such as to treat headaches, shock, and upset. Hold essential oil–infused tissue in cupped hands, one hand as the base, the other cupped over the palm of this hand, forming an enclosed receptacle for the tissue (thus temporarily containing the evaporating vapors), leaving a small inhaling gap between the thumb and forefinger of the upper hand. Inhale vaporizing fragrances through the gap. *Wash your hands when this exercise is finished* to remove excess essential oil that may have transferred from the tissue to your hands or fingers.

Indications
Use for:

+ Anxiety and depression (mild)
+ Chest infections
+ Colds and flu
+ Headaches
+ Immune support (antimicrobial, anti-infectious, antiviral)
+ Improving or reinforcing memory retention
+ Improving respiration
+ Insomnia
+ Mental clarity (to clear head and thoughts)
+ Psycho-emotional moods and conditions—for example, for grief, joy, loss, nervousness, or pleasure, or to balance, calm, invigorate, sedate, or uplift
+ Shock and upset
+ Sinus congestion
+ Sore throat
+ Stress and stress-related conditions

STEAM INHALATION

Another mode of therapeutic inhalation, steam is a great method for clearing the sinuses, relieving sore throats and chest infections, and decongesting the lungs. It also opens and aids cleansing of facial pores; it is a refreshing facial sauna!

Method
You will need a kettle (or pan), water, a heat-proof bowl, tissues, essential oils, and a large towel. Before commencing, ensure that your equipment is placed in a safe position, away from pets and children, and on a stable surface. Heat the water in the kettle to boiling. Very carefully pour the hot water into the bowl. Allow the water to cool slightly (essential oils will vaporize too rapidly otherwise). Add 2 to

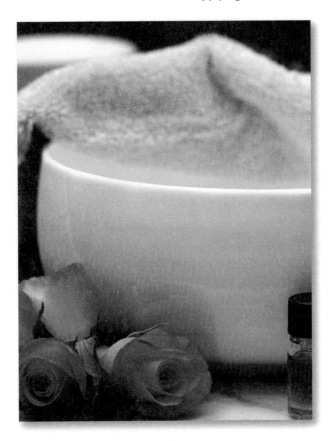

4 drops of your selected essential oil or blend of essential oils to the water.

Cover your head and the bowl with the large towel to contain the rising essential oil–infused steam vapors. **Close your eyes.** Breathe the vapors in through your nose and exhale through your mouth for a few minutes. Remove the towel (come up for air). Replenish the water and essential oils if necessary and repeat the exercise two or three times.

Stop immediately if you experience any irritation or feel dizzy. Essential oils will irritate the mucous membranes to a certain degree; use moderately and do not exceed the above dose. Caution must be applied and the dose reduced if the recipient has sensitivities, asthma, or epilepsy (use half the above dose—1 to 2 drops of essential oil).

Indications

Use for:

+ Anxiety and depression (mild)
+ Chest or bronchial infections or conditions
+ Colds and flu
+ Headaches
+ Immune support (antimicrobial, anti-infectious, antiviral)
+ Improving respiration
+ Insomnia
+ Loosening and/or encouraging release of mucus (expectorant)
+ Mental clarity (to clear head and thoughts)
+ Psycho-emotional moods and conditions—for example, for grief, joy, loss, nervousness, or pleasure, or to balance, calm, invigorate, sedate, or uplift
+ Sinus congestion
+ Skin care: opening and cleansing pores; acne and oily skin; revitalizing and rejuvenating the facial/neck skin (rinse with cool water and/or witch hazel after steam inhalation procedure to close pores)
+ Sore throat
+ Stress and stress-related conditions

ENVIRONMENTAL ROOM VAPORIZERS AND DIFFUSERS

Candle-lit burners are a very popular way of diffusing essential oils and they do create a lovely ambience. However, care must be taken when using this method. For example, always ensure that the candle is extinguished before leaving the burner unattended, keep out of the reach of children, and so on.

Electric steam diffusers have improved by leaps and bounds in terms of their design and are becoming increasingly popular, especially as they are safer to use (although caution must still be applied). They tend to dispense the essential oil–infused steam more rapidly and further into the atmosphere of a room and seem to maintain the integrity of the fragrance better than other methods of diffusion.

Most essential oils can be diffused in either way. However, essential oils extracted from fruits (for example, mandarin and lime), woods (for example, sandalwood, cedarwood, cypress, and pine), flowers (for example, ylang ylang, orange blossom, and of course rose), and resins (such as frankincense and myrrh), to name just a few examples, are especially refreshing, pleasant, and tenacious and can be combined to make lovely blends. Rose otto essential oil is extremely expensive. Rose absolute, though, is less so. Either can be purchased in a 5% mix usually blended in jojoba oil. Both the absolute and otto are intensely perfumed, so using a very small amount is still very effective.

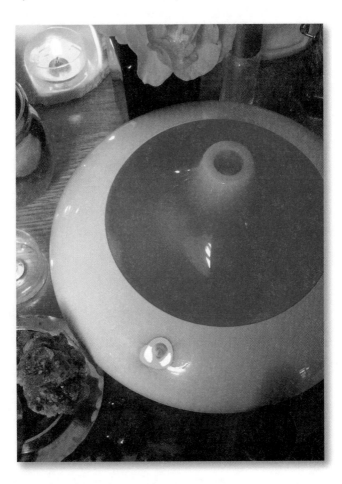

Remember, scent preference is very personal and what one person may really like, another person may not, so when you diffuse essential oils in a communal area, be mindful that the essential oils you choose are agreeable.

The sense of smell soon becomes saturated; the brain stops acknowledging smells after a short period of time, even though they may still be present. However, upon leaving and returning to a room, the scent should be able to be detected again; this may be a good indication of whether the essential oils need replenishing.

Electric Fan or Steam Diffuser Method

These diffusers usually come with instructions regarding appropriate operation and use. Add 6 to 8 drops of an essential oil or essential oil blend. Replenish as necessary. Rather than leaving the diffuser on constantly, use in short bursts at convenient times.

Candle-Lit Diffuser Method

Add water to the bowl. Add 6 to 8 drops of essential oil or essential oil blend. Light the candle. Replenish as necessary. Candle-lit diffusers with deep water bowls are preferable (to avoid rapid drying out). Do not allow water to dry out (keep a small jug of water at hand to replenish).

Do not leave unattended; ensure that the candle is extinguished before leaving it unattended. Place in a safe, stable position, where it cannot be knocked over or touched by children or pets.

Indications

Use for:

+ Aesthetic (environmental) perfumes
+ Antianxiety
+ Antidepressant
+ Calming
+ Improving and/or supporting mood and emotion
+ Improving or creating a particular ambience or theme

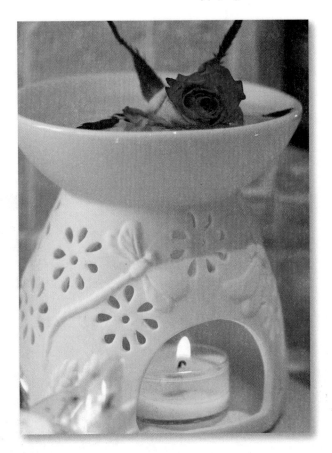

+ Insomnia
+ Masking unpleasant odors
+ Reducing or combating airborne microbes
+ Reducing restlessness and agitation (calming, improving mood and emotion)
+ Stress and stress-related conditions
+ Uplifting

RESIN BURNERS

Resin is collected from incisions in the bark or stem of a tree or plant (for example, frankincense, myrrh, or galbanum) and then dried. It can be heated to release the essential oil contained within.

Terra-cotta resin burners do not conduct heat as rapidly as metal ones so are preferable in terms of safe handling, but they must be placed in a safe, stable position, where they cannot be knocked over. Metal resin burners (used, for example, in religious ceremonies) provide ornate cage-like containers, which allow the essential oil–infused smoke to permeate through holes in the structure, and are suspended on a chain so the container can safely be handled or moved once the resin is heated.

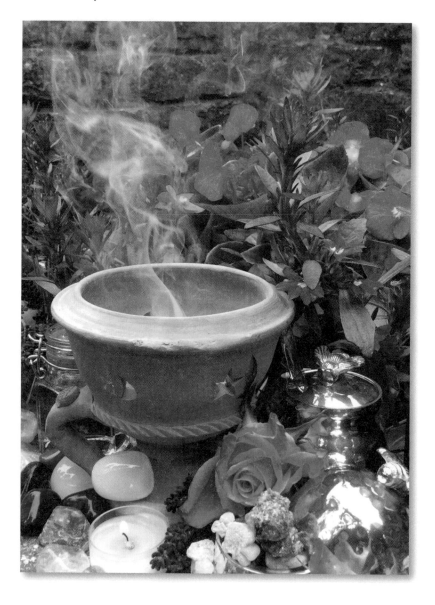

Method

A small, flat piece of charcoal, held firmly with long-handled pincers or tweezers, is lit; once the charcoal sparks, it will rapidly heat. Still using the tweezers, the burning charcoal is placed within the bowl of the container and a small piece of resin is placed on top of it. As the charcoal heats the resin, the resin begins to smoke as it melts and disintegrates; the essential oil is carried within the smoke that infuses into the surrounding atmosphere.

Do not leave the resin burner unattended once lit. Always ensure that the charcoal and resin have burned out. Once finished with, douse with water to extinguish if still burning. Place the container in a safe position where it cannot be accidently knocked over or touched by children or pets.

Indications

Use for:

+ Aesthetics
+ Improving and/or supporting mood and emotion
+ Improving or creating a particular ambience or theme
+ Masking unpleasant odors
+ Meditation

BATHS

Essential oils can be used in the bath for therapeutic purposes as well as for relaxation. When applied in a bath, essential oils are usually absorbed via inhalation of fragrance-infused steam, rather than via the epidermis (skin). Although wetting and soaking the skin with warm water may assist epidermal absorption, hot or warm baths tend to encourage perspiration (excretion) rather than absorption. Water is also drying to the skin; dispensing essential oil in an oily or fatty carrier medium helps form a barrier, which may prevent essential oil irritation and reduce the drying effect of water.

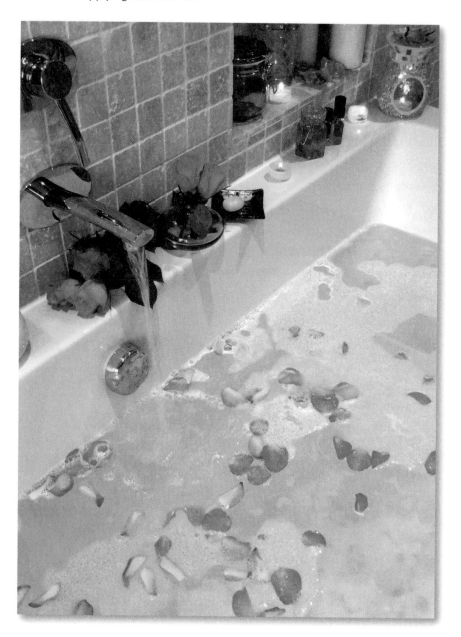

Method

Fill the bath with water, and then, just before getting in, add 6 to 8 drops of essential oil or an essential oil blend dispersed in 20 ml of vegetable oil. Do not use essential oils neat in the bath (water and heat exacerbate the drying and potential irritant effect of essential oils). When dispensing essential oils in vegetable oil into the bath for children, the frail, or very elderly, **be mindful that vegetable oil will make the bath slippery.** Apply essential oils in reduced quantity for children and the elderly. Do not leave children unattended in a bath. To maximize benefit, close windows and doors.

Caution! The following essential oils should *not* be used in the bath: basil, cinnamon, clove, peppermint, and thyme. There is a high risk that these essential oils will cause skin irritation, and peppermint essential oil reduces body temperature.

Indications
Use for:
+ Antidepressant effects
+ Calming restlessness and agitation
+ Improving mood and emotion
+ Insomnia (bathing before bedtime)
+ Relaxation
+ Respiratory conditions, including colds and flu
+ Stress and stress-related conditions
+ Superficial skin conditions
+ Uplifting

SELF-MASSAGE

Self-massage is a wonderful way to nurture yourself. Any movement and stimulation of soft tissue improves circulation and lymphatic drainage. Rhythmic movements and gentle pressure also aid muscle relaxation. Touch is also self-comforting.

Self-massage can be done after a bath or shower, when your skin is warm, clean, and hydrated, using lotion or vegetable oil as a lubricating medium. Adding essential oils to your carrier medium instills further benefits.

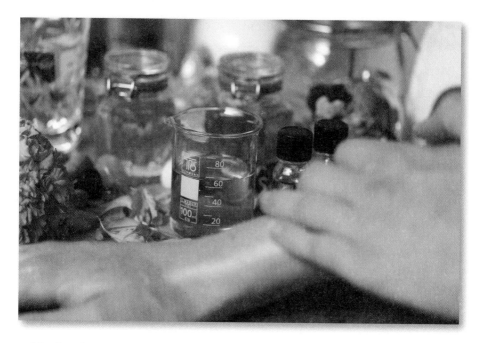

Method

Add 4 to 6 drops of your selected essential oil or essential oil blend to your chosen carrier medium, which should be contained in a small dish or pouring jug. Place the containing vessel on a small saucer to catch drips and spills.

Pour a small amount of the oil mixture into the palm of your hand, then stroke (effleurage) the oil over the area to be massaged.

With the flat of your hand (palms, fingers, and thumbs), apply firm rhythmic stroking and circular movements to your limbs, abdomen, buttocks, shoulders, neck, and face. Gently pick up and squeeze your skin and soft tissue (the fleshy-muscly areas of your body, such as the upper arms, legs, thighs, and buttocks), applying a rhythmic motion.

Working from feet to head tends to be stimulating and thus is a good method for morning massage; working from head to feet is sedating/relaxing and thus appropriate for evening time.

Do not massage over bruises, cuts, or damaged skin.

Indications

Use for:

+ Aiding alertness (morning) and restfulness (evening)
+ Calming
+ Lubricating, softening, and moisturizing skin
+ Relaxation
+ Self-empowerment
+ Soothing
+ Stimulating circulatory and lymphatic systems
+ Stimulating endocrine glands and the release of hormones
+ Stimulating the nervous system via nerve endings in the skin
+ Stress and stress-related conditions
+ Supporting detoxification via the epidermis
+ Supporting feelings of value, self-worth, and self-esteem
+ Supporting the immune system
+ Uplifting

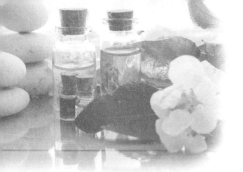

4

Complementary Wellness Techniques

Relaxation, Exercise, and Nutrition

Alongside essential oils and mindfulness, team players in the wellness management toolbox that may support individuals in maintaining their locus of control include, among others, sufficient rest and more general relaxation techniques, exercise, and nutrition.

RELAXATION AND EXERCISE: FINDING A HEALTHY BALANCE

Balance is key to maintaining a healthy lifestyle: the right measure of everything in moderation—movement and stillness, work and rest, eating and fasting. Our body and brain operate in fluctuating rhythmic cycles.

The *circadian rhythm* operates in a twenty-four-hour cycle, which is stimulated by sunlight and darkness. It influences bodily functions such as digestion, bowel movements, and sleep patterns. These functions are optimized at certain times during the twenty-four-hour daytime–nighttime cycle

The *ultradian rhythm* is linked to the 90- to 120-minute brain-wave frequency cycle. The brain is more active than any other organ or muscle in the body, so naturally it tires more quickly. This means it can only sustain intense activity in bursts. The brain automatically switches from the left (rational, problem solving) hemisphere to the right (creative, intuitive) hemisphere—from active to passive mode—to enable it to recover. This cycle also continues during sleep; hence we have deep-sleep and dreaming phases. Thus, our focus and attention peaks and wanes throughout the day. We can only maintain attention for between 90 and 120 minutes before our brain tires and needs to switch modes while it restores.

Our body functions and performs best when it moves freely through regular, balanced, rhythmic cycles of activity and rest. However, the demands of modern life often appear to be at odds with these natural rhythms. Since the industrial revolution, our activity has become mechanized—rather than being liberated from heavy toil by the invention of machinery, it seems we have become slaves in a different sense. Instead of doing less, we are expected to do more. Even our leisure time is consumed by things we *must do*. Where our ancestors spent just a few hours a day hunting and gathering and tending to daily needs, we now find ourselves working around the clock: twenty-four-hour shopping, ten-hour shifts, jobs that have us either sitting for hours in the same sedentary position in front of a computer or a machine or constantly on our feet repeating the same movement or action again and again. Consequently, we are more likely to be distracted, disjointed, and disconnected from our natural state of *being*. This is a recipe for stress, injury, illness, and dis-ease.

We each have our own *way of being:* sitting around the campfire, sharing stories, playing music and dancing, moving our bodies in flow, creating beautiful artwork, simply observing and appreciating the daily and seasonal rhythm of nature. By being aware and proactive, we can manage our own *balance.* By deliberately engaging in exercise (active) and relaxation (passive), for example, especially if we are able to respond in sync with our brain's ultradian rhythm, we help our body restore and retain its natural rhythm and equilibrium.

There are two modes of exercise. One stretches and gently tones muscles and ligaments; improves flexibility, joint movement, core stability, posture, and deportment; and assists the flow and function of internal systems and organs. Examples include yoga, gentle Pilates, and postural awareness and correction techniques such as the Alexander technique and Feldenkrais method. This mode of exercise also aids the body in warming up before more rigorous exercise or sports activities and prevents strain or damage to ligaments, joints, and muscles. The second mode of exercise is more strenuous and involves sustained cardiovascular stimulation; strengthens muscles, including the heart; and improves coordination and stamina. Examples include running and vigorous walking, climbing, swimming, sports activities, dancing, and martial arts, among others.

All exercise improves circulatory, digestive, and metabolic function; increases the elimination of wastes; strengthens muscles and improves mobility; and stimulates the activation of dopamine, serotonin, oxytocin, and endorphins (the happiness neurotransmitters!).

Relaxation stimulates the parasympathetic nervous system (the "rest and digest" system) and also involves two modes. One includes focused and deep relaxation and stillness techniques, such as meditation, visualization, and conscious calming techniques—for example, muscle relaxation, chanting and prayer, and listening to music or sounds like a flowing river or the sea ebbing and flowing on a shore. The other mode involves creative activities such as painting, drawing, and other creative hobbies such as reading for pleasure, walking in nature, and so on.

Both exercise and relaxation improve the quality of sleep, during which time the body can rest, recuperate, and restore. Other benefits include:

+ Improved immune function
+ Improved energy levels
+ Improved circulation
+ Improved oxygen intake and cellular respiration
+ Decreased risk of heart attack and stroke

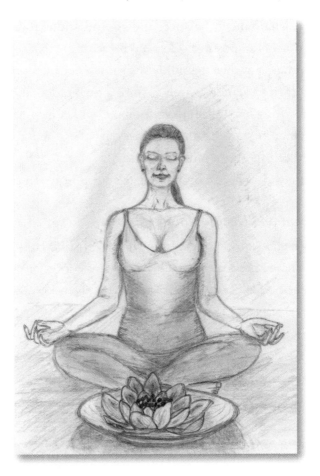

+ Lower blood pressure
+ Protection from mental health problems
+ Improved memory and learning capacity
+ Improved concentration
+ Clearer thinking
+ Better coping mechanisms and skills
+ Improved self-esteem

EXERCISE AND MOBILITY PRACTICES

Stretching and core stability exercises strengthen muscles that support the spine, lower back, and abdomen; improve suppleness and flexibility for improved movement, balance, and coordination; and correct and maintain optimum posture. Correct breathing—that is, using the diaphragm muscle rather than only the muscles of the upper chest—is important during exercise as well as during meditation and relaxation. Correct breathing maximizes oxygen intake, which helps the body and muscles maintain stamina and improves alertness and concentration (oxygenated cells perform more efficiently).

Here is a way to check and modulate your posture and breathing.

◊ Alignment and Deep Breathing Exercise

1. Lie down on your back with your head resting on a small cushion or pillow.

2. Relax your muscles and ensure that your spine is in a neutral position: There are three natural curves in the spine—one in the neck, one in the upper back, and one in the lower back. To check and correct your spine's natural alignment, place one hand on each hip. Gently move your pelvis up and down as far as you comfortably can, finding the position between these two extremes, somewhere in the middle. Hold this position. This should then align the rest of your spine according to its natural curvature.

3. Maintaining this alignment, place one hand on your stomach and one hand on your chest. As you breathe in and out, both hands should move up and down as your abdomen and chest rise and fall with each breath cycle. With shallow breathing your upper chest and shoulders will move—your shoulders should *not* move when you breathe correctly.

4. Keep practicing this alignment and deep breathing until you are comfortable with it and it feels natural. You will then be more able and inclined to maintain this alignment during exercise and other activities.

5. Once you have practiced this lying down, you can also try it in a standing position: Imagine a thread gently pulling you forward from your stomach or solar plexus and, at the same time, another thread gently pulling you up from the top of your head. Hold this position and consciously relax all muscles not required to maintain this stance. Then, in this position of alignment, practice the deep breathing routine.

Exercise and Mobility Practices

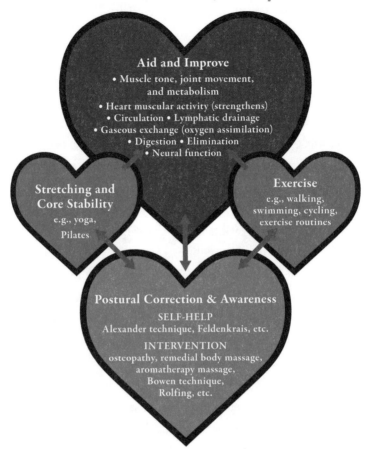

It is helpful to get in the habit of checking and correcting your posture and breathing before commencing exercise or relaxation (or formal meditation). Throughout the day you can also gently return to optimal postural alignment when you notice that you are slouching. Slouching, while it seems comfortable, actually expends more energy as your muscles work harder to keep you upright against the pull of gravity. Slouching also compresses and adds pressure to internal organs.

Vigorous exercise should only be carried out once you have warmed up and stretched your muscles and ligaments. Yoga and Pilates provide very useful warm-up stretching postures and movements. Yoga also provides a safe and effective method of gentle exercise for those who are unable to perform vigorous exercise or activity.

There are many ways of including exercise in your daily life without going to the gym—and they can be fun! Take the stairs instead of the elevator. Walk or bike to work. Swim. Dance. Clean the house or the car (thinking of it as an exercise rather than a chore). Create a standing desk or table to reduce the time you spend sitting. Instead of meeting for coffee, meet for a "walk and talk." If you have to work seated at a desk, stand up and go for a short walk or perform a few simple stretching exercises every hour. The key is to be active in as many ways as possible as often as you can.

Remember that relaxation is not the same as being sedentary and inactive. Relaxation involves deliberate action. Just as exercise can be undertaken in short bursts interspersed throughout the day, so too can concerted relaxation.

The following practices focus on postural alignment, muscle and ligament flexibility, and optimum movement and mobility.

Yoga

An ancient Hindu spiritual and ascetic discipline originating in India 5,000 to 6,000 years ago, yoga was introduced to the West in the nineteenth century. Here it is mainly practiced for health and relaxation. It involves simple meditation, breath control, and performance of a series of specific body postures. Yoga encompasses a wide variety of practices, and two of the most well-known styles are hatha and ashtanga. Hatha yoga focuses on physical and mental strength-building exercises. Ashtanga yoga involves systemic exercises and self-development techniques for body, mind, and spirit. Yoga improves flexibility and balance and strengthens the lower body.

Pilates

A system of exercises devised by and named after Joseph Pilates (1883–1967), this practice was designed to improve physical strength, flexibility, and posture and to enhance mental awareness, with an emphasis on postural alignment, breathing, developing a strong core, and improving coordination and balance. Exercises include stretching and strengthening techniques, which involve mat work and the use of specially designed apparatus.

Alexander Technique

An educational process, designed and named after its creator, Frederick Matthias Alexander (1869–1955), this technique was devised to retrain habitual patterns of movement and posture to ensure minimum effort and strain and support physical well-being. Training involves guided modeling and passive retraining, the aim of which is to break habits and support effortless movement and flow.

Feldenkrais

The goal of this exercise therapy, devised and named after Moshe Feldenkrais (1904–1984), is to reeducate the nervous system and improve motor ability to allow the body to move and function more efficiently and comfortably. The practitioner directs attention to habitual inefficient or strained patterns of movement. Then, using gentle, slow, repeated movements, the practitioner guides the recipient in applying new patterns and aids them in retraining, encouraging, and allowing this new pattern of movement to begin to feel normal. These movements may be performed by the practitioner (passive) or performed by the recipient (active). The aim is to move from a position of mere function to functioning *well*, without pain or restriction of movement.

Bowen

This very subtle, gentle manipulation therapy, devised by Thomas Ambrose Bowen (1916–1982), works on the soft connective tissue (fascia) of the body and relies on stimulating a neural response within the brain. Treatment consists of applying a sequence of small "moves," which typically involve gentle rolling motions, using the thumb and forefinger, along the muscles, tendons, and fascia, followed by pauses (a significant feature of this treatment) that apparently allow the body to reset itself. These moves are designed to stimulate the tissue and nerve pathways, creating a focus for the brain. Recipients remain fully clothed during this procedure. Results are not always immediate but can manifest or become apparent days after treatment.

Rolfing

A deep tissue technique of soft tissue manipulation aimed at realigning the body and optimizing posture in a way that minimizes and reduces the pull of gravity, this system was devised by and named after Ida Rolf (1896–1979). Rolf believed that the human body's energy field benefits from being aligned with the Earth's gravitational field. Rolfing involves the use of a combination of active and passive, deep and superficial movements that stretch the fascia. It is sometimes painful. Rolfing is delivered as a progression of treatments: the first three focus on superficial tissues, the next four on deeper tissues, and the final treatments address the whole body. Treatments are aimed at the reduction of muscular and psychic pain and realignment of the body in accord with the pull of gravity to improve and facilitate easier movement.

Osteopathy

This system is based on the principle that the well-being of the individual is influenced by the smooth functioning, alignment, and coordination of muscles, ligaments, connective tissue (fascia), and bones (particularly bones of the spine). Treatment involves manipulation, stretching, and massage of muscle tissue and realignment of bones. The aim of treatment is to increase mobility of joints, relieve muscle tension, enhance blood supply to tissues, and realign the spine to improve skeletal posture and alleviate and prevent muscle strain, thus also allowing the body's internal organs and systems to function more efficiently.

Remedial Massage

This dynamic, deep tissue massage involves assessment and treatment of muscles, tendons, ligaments, and connective tissue to manage pain and injury and assist in rehabilitation. Alongside deep tissue massage, other appropriate massage techniques are applied depending on the needs of the recipient. The aim of treatment is to restore and maximize the body's ability to function efficiently in a pain-free state.

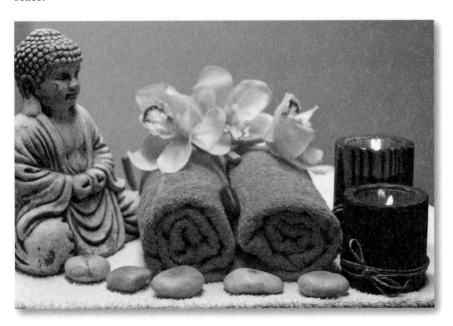

Aromatherapy Massage

Aromatherapy massage is a deeply relaxing massage that incorporates flowing movements and gentle manipulation of muscles and soft tissue. An eclectic mix of techniques is often applied (for instance, gentle acupressure and Swedish massage) depending on need and the therapist's style and approach. The main aim of aromatherapy massage is to achieve deep relaxation, relieve muscle tension, and warm surface tissue and improve circulation to assist absorption of essential oils into the epidermis (skin), the soft tissue below the surface, and the circulatory system.

GUIDELINES FOR OPTIMAL NUTRITION

What we eat is an essential determining factor for our overall health, but how and when we eat are also important. It is advisable to eat during periods of relaxation. Do not eat on the go. Of course, another important factor affecting efficient assimilation of nutrients is to *enjoy your food*. If you are feeling anxious, eat little and often to maintain your blood sugar levels (low blood sugar exacerbates feelings of anxiety), and include carbohydrates that release energy slowly, such as oats and other whole grains, in your diet. Do not skip meals; eat well at breakfast, moderately at lunch and suppertime (do not eat heavy meals in the evening). Drink plenty of water in between meals.

Eat a varied range of fresh foods to ensure intake of vital nutrients (proteins, carbohydrates, fats, vitamins, minerals, and trace elements). A balanced diet consists of:

+ Fruit and vegetables (35%)
+ Carbohydrates: rice and grains, cereals, pasta, bread (35%)
+ Proteins: soya, legumes and grains, certain vegetables, meat, fish, and eggs (15%)
+ Dairy: milk, cheese (10%; NB: dairy is not essential and can be substituted with plant foods)
+ Foods containing non-hydrogenated fats and natural, unprocessed sugars (5%)

It is not necessary to eat meat; plants do provide a rich source of protein and iron, among other vital nutrients (though the quality of the soil in which vegetables and grains are grown affects the mineral and trace element content of the plant). A vegetarian diet results in a greatly reduced carbon footprint (farming and food production) compared to a diet high in meat and animal products, a vegan diet even less.[1] This does not mean that meat should be eliminated (this is a personal choice), only that it should be eaten in moderation and sourced from ethical, environmentally friendly suppliers.

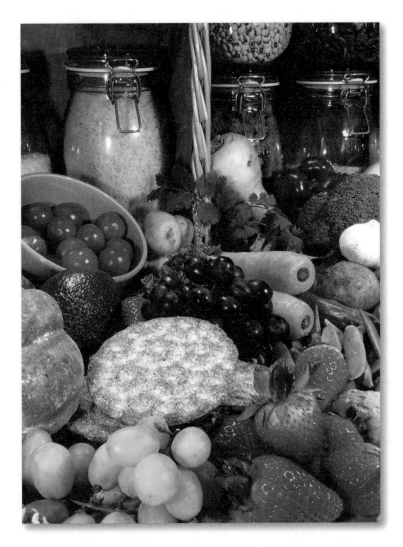

Nutritional Values of Food

The food chart on the following pages will enable you to select foods rich in appropriate nutrients to balance your diet. The foods listed here provide the macronutrients (protein, carbohydrate, fat, water), micronutrients (vitamins, minerals, and trace elements), and fiber required for healthy digestion. Vitamins are presented first, alphabetically, followed by macrominerals and trace minerals, which are presented in general order of quantity (beginning with those minerals the body requires the largest quantity of).

VITAMINS AND MINERALS REQUIRED BY THE BODY TO SUSTAIN HEALTHY FUNCTION

VITAMINS AND MINERALS	FOOD SOURCES OF VITAL NUTRIENTS	SYMPTOMS OF NUTRIENT DEFICIENCY
Vitamin A *(Supports immune system, cell growth, vision)*	*Retinoids (animal sources)* Fish, liver Eggs, milk, butter, cheese, dairy products *Beta-carotene (vegetable sources)* Soybeans Carrots, yams, sweet potatoes, pumpkin, other yellow vegetables; apricots, peaches, papaya, cantaloupe	Red itchy eyes, night blindness, vision difficulties in dim light, sensitivity to bright light; dry rough skin; a predisposition to colds and infection; broken tooth enamel; kidney stones; allergies
Vitamin B1 Thiamine *(Rapidly destroyed by heat; aids assimilation of carbohydrates, helps convert blood sugar into energy; aids breakdown of proteins and carbohydrates, memory function, mucous membrane integrity, development of myelin sheaths and nerve function)*	Liver Milk, egg yolk Legumes (beans, peas, lentils, peanuts, etc.) Rice, bran and raw germ of cereals, brewer's yeast, molasses Green leafy vegetables, yellow vegetables, fruit	Nervous disorders: neurosis, neurasthenia (nervous exhaustion), irritability, sensitivity to noise, loss of morale, fear, anxiety, confusion; low thyroid functions; appetite loss; heart palpitations
Vitamin B2 Riboflavin *(Concerned with carbohydrate and protein metabolism, skin development and function, lining of intestinal tract and blood cells)*	Liver, fish roe Eggs, milk, dairy products Brewer's yeast Green leafy vegetables	Mouth and lip lesions, tongue inflammation, sensation of sand in eyes, red itchy eyes, cataracts; scaly skin on face, impairment of red blood cell formation leading to anemia and heart disease; dental problems; congenital birth defects

VITAMINS AND MINERALS	FOOD SOURCES OF VITAL NUTRIENTS	SYMPTOMS OF NUTRIENT DEFICIENCY
Vitamin B3 Niacin *(Associated with energy release in cells; aids body utilization of carbohydrates, proteins, and fatty acids to create energy; works with other B vitamins to convert macronutrients into energy)*	Liver Fish Eggs Brewer's yeast, raw wheat germ, peanut butter Avocados, dried fruits (e.g., dates, figs, prunes)	Pellagra (disease that may result in scaly skin, diarrhea, mental disorders); indigestion, fatigue, mouth disorders, loss of sense of humor, headaches, depression, dementia, schizophrenia
Vitamin B5 Pantothenic acid *(Associated with amino acid metabolism; aids efficient utilization of carbohydrates, proteins, and lipids; skin regeneration)*	Meat, organ meat (liver, kidney) Cod roe, royal jelly Raw wheat germ, whole grains, beans, brewer's yeast, molasses, nuts	Mental stress, irritability, depression, hypoglycemia, allergies, arthritis, gastric conditions (ulcers, indigestion, and constipation), fatigue, graying hair, skin disorders
Vitamin B6 Pyridoxine *(Associated with supporting proper function of carbohydrates and lipids, amino acid metabolism, the production of antibodies)*	Liver, kidney Eggs, milk Peas, beans, soybeans Brewer's yeast, raw wheat germ, molasses Cabbage	Skin striations, linear nail ridges, inability to tan, sensitivity to sun, tongue inflammation, cracks around lips, numbness of hands and feet, convulsions in children, depression, tremors and seizures (as in Parkinsonism and epilepsy), hypoglycemia, diabetes, appetite loss, high cholesterol, kidney stones, arthritis, allergies, anemia, edema, poor dream recall
Vitamin B7 Biotin (also known as vitamin H) *(Coenzyme, synthesized by microbes in intestine; associated with metabolism of carbohydrates; supports healthy skin, digestive tract, nerves, metabolism, cell formation and regeneration)*	Liver Egg yolk, milk Nuts Brewer's yeast, brown rice Fruits, tomatoes	Eczema, dermatitis, lack of appetite, fatigue, muscle aches and pains

VITAMINS AND MINERALS	FOOD SOURCES OF VITAL NUTRIENTS	SYMPTOMS OF NUTRIENT DEFICIENCY
Vitamin B9 Folate Folic Acid *(Aids healthy development of cells, key to the synthesis of nucleic acid)*	Liver, kidney Egg yolks Torula yeast, beans Green leafy vegetables, carrots, cantaloupe, pumpkin, avocados	Megaloblastic anemia, depression, psychosis, epileptic fits, lack of appetite, sore tongue, digestive disturbances
Vitamin B12 Cyanocobalamin *(Essential for maintenance of myelin, the nervous system and spinal cord nerves, production of elements of DNA, red blood cells, regeneration of bone marrow and lining of the gastrointestinal and respiratory tracts, and melatonin production)*	Liver, kidney, meat Eggs, dairy products Fermented liquors, yeast	Severe: pernicious anemia; mild: sore tongue, shortness of breath, heart palpitations, apathy, weakness, loss of coordination, impaired memory, senile dementia, sharp mood swings
Vitamin B15 Pangamic acid *(Antioxidant, stimulates cellular respiration and prevents cellular oxidization, aids the formation of amino acids, enhances liver function, mild stimulant of endocrine and nervous system; not an essential vitamin)*	Brewer's yeast Brown rice, whole grains Pumpkin seeds Sesame seeds	Reduced oxygenation of cells, leading to fatigue, low levels of fitness, premature aging, heart disease, glandular and nervous conditions
Vitamin C Ascorbic acid *(Antioxidant; keeps cholesterol in bloodstream from oxidizing; associated with metabolism of protein; important factor in collagen production; easily damaged by heat)*	Whole citrus fruits and juices (fresh), black currants, elderberries, rose hips Peppers, broccoli, tomatoes, cabbage, green leafy vegetables, melons, yams, potatoes (raw to semi-cooked)	Susceptibility to colds, infections and allergies, bleeding or inflamed gums, defective teeth; broken capillaries and subskin hemorrhages, strokes, anemia, skin wrinkles, loss of appetite, fatigue, nervousness, anxiety, depression, impaired healing of wounds

VITAMINS AND MINERALS	FOOD SOURCES OF VITAL NUTRIENTS	SYMPTOMS OF NUTRIENT DEFICIENCY
Choline *(Similar to the B vitamins; made in the liver from components in the foods listed; supports nervous system)*	Brains, liver Egg yolks Brewer's yeast, raw wheat germ Green leafy vegetables	Fatty degeneration of liver, nephritis (kidney disease), gallstones, intolerance of fats (gallbladder syndrome), nerve-muscle diseases, high cholesterol, atherosclerosis, hypertension
Vitamin D *(Metabolized via sun exposure on skin and foods listed; regulates calcium and phosphorus metabolism, important factor for healthy bones and teeth)*	Fish liver oil, sardines, herring, salmon, tuna Fortified milk, eggs, butter, cheese	Soft and porous bones and teeth, leading to rickets, tooth decay, or osteoporosis; fatigue, arthritis, myopia (shortsightedness)
Vitamin E *(Antioxidant, important for cell membrane integrity; prevents catabolism of polyunsaturated fats; protects artery walls, and myelin sheaths surrounding nerves)*	Egg yolks, butter, milk Nuts Soybeans, whole grains and cereals Raw wheat germ and wheat germ oil, vegetable oils Leafy green vegetables	Fatigue, premature aging, infertility, sterility, miscarriage, muscular dystrophy, hemolytic anemia, coronary heart disease, thrombosis, swollen and inflamed veins, lameness due to poor circulation (nephritis), degeneration of sex glands (testes, prostate), poor healing of wounds and burns
Inositol *(Made from glucose; present in all living cells)*	Liver, kidney, brains Brewer's yeast, wheat germ Molasses, peanut butter Cantaloupe	Hypertension, high cholesterol levels, atherosclerosis, dermatitis, constipation, hair loss **NOTE:** diabetics and alcohol and coffee drinkers overexcrete inositol and therefore need supplements to prevent deficiency

VITAMINS AND MINERALS	FOOD SOURCES OF VITAL NUTRIENTS	SYMPTOMS OF NUTRIENT DEFICIENCY
Vitamin K *(Aids blood clotting/ coagulation and synthesis of proteins, binds calcium in bones; directly involved in photosynthesis in plants)*	Liver Fish, fish liver oil Egg yolks, yogurt, buttermilk Alfalfa, green leafy vegetables, kelp Safflower and soybean oil	Delayed blood clotting, hemorrhages, lack of blood platelets; deficiency usually caused by defect in metabolism or a malfunction of the liver, colitis, or celiac disease (celiac disease is caused by intestinal intolerance to gluten, a protein found in wheat, rye, and barley)
Vitamin P Flavonoids *(A by-product of plant metabolism; reduces blood sugar and lipids; improves insulin resistance; anti-inflammatory; aids absorption of iron)*	Citrus fruits (especially the pith and rind), grapes, plums, black currants, apricots, buckwheat leaves, cherries, rose hips	Bruising
MACROMINERALS		
Potassium (K) *(Involved in intracellular activity, contraction of muscles, transmission of nerve impulses, maintenance of the electrolyte balance in the body)*	Citrus fruits, green leafy vegetables, bananas, potatoes, tomatoes, pineapple, avocados, nuts (widely distributed in all foods)	Edema, hypertension, irregular heartbeat, nervousness, fatigue, arthritis
Sodium (Na) *(Works with potassium ions to build up charges on cell membranes, assisting transmission of nerve impulses)*	Meats Shellfish Eggs, milk, enriched bread Sea salt, soy sauce, tamari Kelp, beets, carrots, chard, dandelion greens	Intestinal gas, weight loss, muscle wasting, fatigue, dehydration NOTE: deficiencies are very uncommon but can be caused by excessive perspiration

VITAMINS AND MINERALS	FOOD SOURCES OF VITAL NUTRIENTS	SYMPTOMS OF NUTRIENT DEFICIENCY
Calcium (Ca) *(Associated with vitamin D and phosphorus in the hardening of bones and teeth; involved in the coagulation of blood and action of muscle contraction)*	Some fish, particularly canned fish Milk, cheese, dairy products Sesame seeds and tahini, soybeans, peanuts, walnuts, sunflower seeds Honey, molasses Green leafy vegetables	Porous and brittle bones, fractures, tooth decay, rickets, nervousness, muscle aches, leg cramps, teeth grinding, skin disorders, loss of pigmentation, cold sores, mouth blisters, excessive menstrual flow, impaired growth
Phosphorus (P) *(Associated with calcium and vitamin D in hardening of bones and teeth; helps maintain the constant composition of the body fluids)*	Meat, liver, kidney Fish Eggs, cheese Nuts and seeds Whole grains, raw wheat germ, oatmeal	Weak bones and teeth, rickets, gum infection and bleeding, arthritis, loss of appetite, muscle weakness
Magnesium (Mg) *(Required for over 300 biochemical reactions of the body; supports growth and maintenance of bones, heart, nerve and muscle function, immune system)*	Nuts (especially almonds), seeds Wheat germ, yellow corn, whole grains (especially brown rice, millet), beans, peas, figs, lemons, grapefruits, apples, green leafy vegetables Coffee Natural supplement—dolomite	Irregular heartbeat and heart attacks, jumpy nerves, weak muscles, convulsions and seizures, prostate enlargement, fatigue, bedwetting, kidney stones
Sulfur (S) *(Supports enzyme reactions and protein synthesis, collagen formation, cell respiration; necessary for maintenance of hair, nails, skin)*	A nonmetallic mineral, abundant in nature and present in every animal and plant cell; present in four amino acids plus thiamine and biotin (B vitamins)	Arthritis, dry hair, brittle nails and rough skin

TRACE MINERALS		
VITAMINS AND MINERALS	**FOOD SOURCES OF VITAL NUTRIENTS**	**SYMPTOMS OF NUTRIENT DEFICIENCY**
Iron (Fe) *(A vital mineral that aids transportation of oxygen around body and is involved in conversion of blood-sugar into energy; a component of hemoglobin; aids maintenance of healthy hair, skin, nails)*	Liver, kidneys, beef, raw clams, oysters Egg yolks Dried beans Oatmeal, molasses Dried peaches, raisins, prunes, green leafy vegetables	Iron deficiency anemia, pallor, weakness, shortness of breath, brittle nails
Zinc (Zn) *(Antioxidant; protects against aging of skin and muscles; supports immune system; supports cell division and growth; vital for brain activity during detection of taste and smell; vital for healthy vision)*	Meat, fish, raw oysters Egg yolks, milk Dried legumes, whole grains Raw wheat germ, brewer's yeast, pumpkin seeds, sunflower seeds, ground mustard seeds Mushrooms	Prostate trouble, sterility, delayed sexual maturation, menstrual irregularities, retarded growth and dwarfism, birth defects such as mental retardation and slow learning, susceptibility to infections and poor wound healing, joint pains, arteriosclerosis and poor circulation, fatigue, lack of appetite, loss of sense of taste and smell, susceptibility to diabetes, allergies, acne, stretch marks, depigmentation (white spots) of nails, offensive perspiration
Manganese (Mn) *(Necessary for bone development and maintenance, proper nerve function, and metabolism; antioxidant; stored in bones, liver, and kidneys)*	Nuts, pumpkin seeds Whole grains, whole wheat, oats, peas Cloves, ginger, tea leaves Green leafy vegetables, especially spinach, watercress, beet greens, peppermint Strawberries, blackberries, bananas Molasses	Low tolerance to carbohydrates, skeletal abnormalities (legs too short or long), loss of muscle condition, convulsions

VITAMINS AND MINERALS	FOOD SOURCES OF VITAL NUTRIENTS	SYMPTOMS OF NUTRIENT DEFICIENCY
Copper (Cu) *(Necessary for producing and storing iron and for healthy function of organs and metabolism; necessary for proper growth, development, and maintenance of bone, connective tissue, brain, heart; involved in formation of red blood cells and synthesis and release of life-sustaining proteins and enzymes)*	Liver, kidney Seafoods, especially shellfish Soybeans, legumes (beans, lentils), whole grains, especially whole wheat and rye Molasses, chocolate Peanuts, pecans Prunes, kale, apples	Anemia, fatigue, shortness of breath, skin depigmentation
Iodine (I) *(Constituent of thyroxine and triiodothyronine; has nutritional relationship with selenium; necessary for healthy function of gastric mucosa, salivary glands, arterial walls, thymus, epidermis, choroid plexus, cerebrospinal fluid, breasts during lactation)*	Shellfish Kelp, seaweeds, onions, strawberries Milk, yogurt, eggs Sea salt	Goiter—characterized by swelling of the thyroid gland in the lower neck; hypothyroidism—symptoms include obesity, dry hair, rapid pulse, heart palpitations, a cold body, constipation, weakness, excessive menstruation, nervousness, low resistance to colds and infections, irritability
Chromium (Cr) *(Aids balance of blood sugar by supporting body's use of insulin; aids metabolism and storage of carbohydrates, fat, and protein)*	Meat, eggs Shellfish, clams Brewer's yeast, molasses, raw wheat germ, rice bran Broccoli, garlic, basil, apples, bananas, green beans	Fatigue, slow growth, obesity, hypertension, high cholesterol levels, impaired glucose metabolism, diabetes

VITAMINS AND MINERALS	FOOD SOURCES OF VITAL NUTRIENTS	SYMPTOMS OF NUTRIENT DEFICIENCY
Fluoride (Fl⁻) *(Essential for mineralization of bones and formation of dental enamel; present in bones, teeth, thyroid gland, skin)*	Seafood Cheese Kelp Fluoridated drinking water, tea Small amounts naturally occur in water, air, plants, animals	Demineralization of bones and teeth, wrinkled skin, lowered resistance to colds and infections, low energy levels
Molybdenum (Mo) *(Stored in the liver, kidneys, glands, bones, tooth enamel; plays important role in normal body functions— protecting cells, creating energy, supporting liver and kidneys to remove waste products; aids in metabolism of fats and carbohydrates and breakdown of certain amino acids)*	Organ meat Milk, cheese, eggs Legumes (lentils, beans, peas), nuts, seeds Whole grain cereals Dark green leafy vegetables, green beans, cucumber	Predisposition to tooth decay, anemia, esophageal cancer, lowered sexual potency (men)

VITAMINS AND MINERALS	FOOD SOURCES OF VITAL NUTRIENTS	SYMPTOMS OF NUTRIENT DEFICIENCY
Selenium (Se) *(Antioxidant, especially when combined with vitamin E; catalyst for production of active thyroid hormone; necessary for proper function of immune system; required for sperm motility)*	Liver Fish—tuna, mackerel, halibut, herring Shellfish—oysters, scallops, lobster Butter Brazil nuts, sunflower seeds Raw wheat germ Brewer's yeast Garlic, onions Whole grains **NOTE:** Selenium is destroyed when foods are processed; a variety of whole, unprocessed foods provides best source of dietary selenium.	Fatigue, susceptibility to infections and disease, premature aging, predisposition to cancer, low sex drive, mood swings
Germanium (Ge) *(Acts against inflammation; balances/ regulates body's ions and removes excess positive ions; strengthens immune system, improves blood circulation, raises oxygen levels, speeds up metabolism of body cells, removes harmful toxins, reduces cholesterol levels)*	Trace amounts in most foods; richer amounts in ginseng, garlic, aloe vera, comfrey, broccoli, celery, mushrooms, rhubarb, tomato juice	Increased susceptibility to the degenerative diseases associated with aging, infection, and immune disorders, heart disease, high cholesterol, arthritis, osteoporosis

VITAMINS AND MINERALS	FOOD SOURCES OF VITAL NUTRIENTS	SYMPTOMS OF NUTRIENT DEFICIENCY
Boron (B) *(Affects the way the body utilizes other minerals— magnesium, phosphorus; increases estrogen levels in postmenopausal women)*	Fruits—apples, peaches, oranges, red grapes, pears, plums, currants, kiwis, sultanas, dates, tomatoes Vegetables—avocado, olives, onion Soybeans, chickpeas, red kidney beans, borlotti beans, lentils Hazelnuts	Calcium loss, bone demineralization, arthritis, low estrogen levels in menopause, reduced growth, abnormal metabolism of calcium and magnesium

Protein

Protein is the collective label applied to identify amino acids. Amino acids are organic compounds that are composed of amine ($-NH2$) and carboxylic acid ($-COOH$). They also have additional amino-acid-specific carbon "side chains," which are attached to a "main chain" or "backbone." Proteins form the second largest component of muscle cells and body tissues; water comprises the largest. There are around 500 known amino acids. However, just twenty-two standard amino acids are required for proper function of the body. Of these, nine are vital (or essential) because they cannot be created from other compounds by the body; they must be ingested (eaten) as food and absorbed. Protein is required by the body for:

Cells: nucleoproteins are found in nucleus of every cell

Enzymes: break down food for absorption; nutrient absorption and waste removal in cells; growth, development, movement, reproduction

Hemoglobin: This iron-rich protein carries oxygen around the body

Myoglobin and elastin: found in muscle fibers

Bones: mainly comprised of protein (plus calcium, magnesium, phosphate)

Hormones: regulation of metabolism

Antibodies: immunity

Keratin: to form nails and hair

The signs and symptoms of protein deficiency are edema, weight loss, thinning or brittle hair, ridges in nails, pale skin, skin rashes, general weakness, slow healing, difficulty sleeping, headaches, and fainting. Other symptoms include crankiness, moodiness, depression, anxiety, lack of energy, and no desire to do things. The following table can be used as a guide to ensure you are getting enough protein.

PROTEIN DAILY REQUIREMENT

AGE GROUP	AMOUNT
Infants aged 1 to 3 years	13 g
Children aged 4 to 8 years	19 g
Children aged 9 to 13 years	34 g
Girls aged 14 to 18 years	46 g
Boys aged 14 to 18 years	52 g
Women aged 19 + years	46 g
Men aged 19 + years	56 g

Two types of proteins are found in food: complete (first class) and incomplete (second class). Complete proteins contain *all* the required amino acids that are necessary to maintain health in one food source. Incomplete proteins, mainly found in vegetables, do not. However, incomplete proteins can be combined to provide a range of amino acids, which ultimately create a complete protein. For example, grains such as wheat, rice, and corn, when combined with legumes such as beans, peas, and lentils, collectively provide sufficient amino acids to form a whole protein. Hummus and pita bread, for example, do the same, as do peanut butter and whole wheat bread, rice and dhal (lentils), and so on. These can be consumed in different meals during the day; they do not need to all be present in one meal.

22 AMINO ACIDS REQUIRED BY
THE BODY FOR PROPER FUNCTION

ESSENTIAL— CANNOT BE MADE WITHIN THE BODY	NON-ESSENTIAL
Histidine	Alanine
Isoleucine	Arginine*
Leucine	Asparagine
Lysine	Aspartic acid
Methionine	Cysteine*
Phenylalanine	Glutamic acid
Threonine	Glutamine*
Tryptophan	Glycine
Valine	Proline*
	Pyrrolysine*
	Selenocysteine*
	Serine*
	Tyrosine*

*Indicates proteins that are essential in some circumstances—for example, in children to support growth

FOOD SOURCES
OF AMINO ACIDS (PROTEIN)

COMPLETE (FIRST CLASS)	**Animal Sources** Meat, fish, eggs, milk, cheese and other milk products except butter **Plant Sources** Quinoa, buckwheat, hempseed, chia, soy, sprouted beans (and vegetable sources below) **Combined Vegetable Sources: Examples** Grains (rice, wheat, corn) + legumes (beans, peas, lentils) Spirulina + grains + nuts
INCOMPLETE (SECOND CLASS)	**Vegetables That Contain Amino Acids (Protein)** Soybeans, lentils, black beans, chickpeas, chai seeds, tofu, pumpkin seeds, sunflower seeds, rolled oats, buckwheat, green peas, almond butter, peanut butter, almonds and other nuts, quinoa, millet, rye grains, wheat, brown rice, corn, flaxseeds, coconut, broccoli, spinach, spirulina, kale, romaine lettuce, mushrooms, artichokes

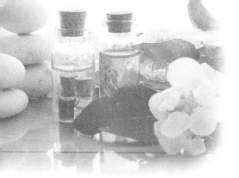

Conclusion

Entering into Your Own Voyage of Discovery

At the epicenter of the storm, there is calm; at the center of chaos, stillness; at the heart of *being*, peace.

Meditation returns consciousness to the peace, stillness, and calm at the epicenter of our being. Remaining mindfully aware, we are present and consciously engaged in the here and now.

Meditation is not a magic wand that waves all our cares away and whisks up our "happily ever after." It may still rain on your wedding day; your flight may still be canceled as you are about to embark on the holiday of a lifetime; you may not win the game or get the promotion you hoped for.

What meditation does is to enable you to stand at the center of each moment and observe, and thus gain a greater sense of awareness of what *is*.

The moment never offers more than we can deal with, yet the outcome of present-centered awareness and meditation is manifold. It's a little bit like rewilding the soul. Left to its own devices, an overplowed and depleted field, abandoned and barren of life after years of repeatedly growing the same crop, will suddenly begin to bloom again as nature magnificently reclaims its territory. In rediscovering our own magnificence, we then notice that life is full of miracles that completely outshine rain on our wedding day.

Essential oils are gifts of nature—one of many manifestations of Earth's nurturing abundance—that provide amazing supportive qualities. They are physiologically protective, restorative, and healing. Observing the scent of essential oils, we are aware of our breathing and, consequently, of the immediacy of the moment. Essential oil molecules instigate various responses within the body, the most significant of which, in terms of meditation, is their influence on the limbic system and their consequential ability to calm, ground, and uplift mood and emotion; aid memory and improve alertness; and inspire a sense of pleasure and joy.

Having completed this book, you are now ready to go on your own voyage of discovery. The basic tenets that underpin the philosophy and practice of mindfulness and meditation presented here lay the groundwork for you to begin to practice, so you can discover for yourself the myriad benefits. Remember, meditation is a proactive process.

Equally, now that you understand the basic nature of essential oils and how they work within the body, you can confidently and safely experiment and discover which oils work best for you as supportive aids to your practice of meditation. For example, you may choose to create a personalized blend of essential oils to diffuse during meditation, perhaps to aid your wakefulness and concentration or to calm your mood. You may also decide to add your blend to jojoba or grapeseed oil to wear as a perfume during the day—to remind you of being in meditation and provide a gentle hint to remain mindfully aware and present as you carry out your daily tasks.

In parting, I leave you with the words of poet Kahlil Gibran:

> *Your daily life is your temple and your religion.*
> *Whenever you enter into it take with you your all.*[1]

Notes

INTRODUCTION

1. Brand, *Revolution,* 129.
2. Burch, "The Mindful Way to Well Being," 1.
3. Quote from ancient Babylonian tablet, found in Tisserand, *Art of Aromatherapy,* 20.
4. Gruner, *Treatise on the Canon,* 233.
5. Culpeper, *English Physitian Enlarged,* 275.
6. All biblical references in the book are quoted from www.biblestudytools .com/kjv.
7. Rudra Vaisnava Sampradaya: Sridhara Swami Commentary, *Srimad Bhagavad-Gita* 15:13. www.bhagavad-gita.org/Gita/verse-15-13.html (accessed May 20, 2018).
8. Tisserand, *Art of Aromatherapy.*

CHAPTER 1.
WHAT IS MINDFULNESS?

1. Mace, *Mindfulness and Mental Health,* 1.
2. Gunaratana, *Beyond Mindfulness,* 1.
3. Mehta, *Holistic Consciousness,* 36.
4. Kabat-Zinn, "Coming to Our Senses," 1.
5. Gunaratana, *Beyond Mindfulness,* 17.
6. Shapiro et al., "Meditation and Positive Psychology," 634.

7. Fromm, *Art of Listening,* 39.

8. Fromm, *Art of Listening,* 180.

9. Rogers, *A Way of Being,* 134.

10. Gunaratana, *Beyond Mindfulness,* 32–34.

11. Mace, *Mindfulness and Mental Health,* 9, 13.

12. Snyder and Lopez, "Mindfulness, Flow, and Spirituality," 243–62.

13. Shapiro et al., "Mindfulness-Based Stress Reduction for Health Care Professionals," 164–76.

14. Gunaratana, *Beyond Mindfulness,* 32–34.

15. Shapiro et al., "Mindfulness-Based Stress Reduction for Health Care Professionals," 164–76.

16. Shapiro et al., "Meditation and Positive Psychology," 634.

17. Rinpoche, "How to Do Mindfulness Meditation."

18. Chambers et al., "Mindful Emotion Regulation," 560–67.

19. Gunaratana, *Beyond Mindfulness,* 32–34.

20. Shapiro et al., "Meditation and Positive Psychology," 634.

21. Mace, *Mindfulness and Mental Health,* 73–74.

22. Kutz et al., "Meditation and Psychotherapy," discussed in Mace, *Mindfulness and Mental Health,* 73–74.

23. Goldin et al., "Mindfulness Meditation Training and Self-Referential Processing in Social Anxiety Disorder," 242–57.

24. Mackenzie et al., "A Brief Mindfulness Based Stress Reduction Intervention for Nurses and Nurse Aides," 105–9.

25. Shapiro et al., "Mindfulness-Based Stress Reduction for Health Care Professionals," 164–76.

26. Wang et al., "Cerebral Blood Flow Changes Associated with Different Meditation Practices and Perceived Depth of Meditation," 60–67.

27. Holzel et al., "Mindfulness Practice Leads to Increases in Regional Brain Gray Matter Density," 36–43.

28. Goldin et al., "Mindfulness Meditation Training and Self-Referential Processing in Social Anxiety Disorder," 242–57.

29. Prem Rawat, "Words of Peace," www.youtube.com/user/wopgyt. Additional quotes of Prem Rawat can be found at www.inspiringquotes.us and at http://theypi.net (accessed May 21, 2018).

30. Shapiro et al., "Mindfulness-Based Stress Reduction for Health Care Professionals," 164–76.

31. Rinpoche, "How to Do Mindfulness Meditation."
32. Rinpoche, "How to Do Mindfulness Meditation."

CHAPTER 2.
ESSENTIAL OILS AS MEDITATION COMPANIONS

1. Tisserand and Young, *Essential Oil Safety,* 5.
2. Lawrence, *Essential Oils 1988–1991,* 187–88.
3. Tisserand and Young, *Essential Oil Safety,* 58.
4. Tisserand and Young, *Essential Oil Safety,* 42.
5. Damian and Damian, *Aromatherapy,* 94, 141–65.
6. Busse et al., "A Synthetic Sandalwood Odorant Induces Wound Healing Process in Human Keratinocytes via Olfactory Receptor OR2AT4," 2823–32; Stone, "Smell Turns Up in Unexpected Places"; Griffin et al., "MOR23 Promotes Muscle Regeneration and Regulates Cell Adhesion and Migration," 649–61; Pluznick et al., "Functional Expression of the Olfactory Signaling System in the Kidney," 2059–64; Spehr et al., "Identification of a Testicular Odorant Receptor Mediating Human Sperm Chemotaxis," 2054–58.
7. Sheppard-Hanger, *Aromatherapy Practitioner Reference Manual,* vol. 2, part 3, Clinical Index, 446.
8. Buchbauer et al., "Fragrance Compounds and Essential Oils with Sedative Effects upon Inhalation," 661.
9. Kovar et al., "Blood Levels of 1,8-cineole and Locomotor Activity of Mice after Inhalation and Oral Administration of Rosemary Oil," 315–18.
10. Moss et al., "Aromas of Rosemary and Lavender Essential Oils Differentially Affect Cognition and Mood in Healthy Adults," 15–38.
11. Moss and Oliver, "Plasma 1,8-cineole Correlates with Cognitive Performance following Exposure to Rosemary Essential Oil Aroma," 103–11.
12. Ilmberger et al., "The Influence of Essential Oils on Human Attention. 1: Alertness," 239–45.
13. Friedmann, "Attention Deficit and Hyperactivity Disorder (ADHD)."
14. Ballard et al., "Aromatherapy as a Safe and Effective Treatment for the Management of Agitation in Severe Dementia," 553–58.
15. Perry, "Aromatherapy for the Treatment of Alzheimer's Disease."

16. Pengelly et al., "Short-Term Study on the Effects of Rosemary on Cognitive Function in an Elderly Population," 10–17.

17. Jimbo et al., "Effect of Aromatherapy on Patients with Alzheimer's Disease," 173–79.

18. Haze et al., "Effects of Fragrance Inhalation on Sympathetic Activity in Normal Adults," 247–53.

19. Chang and Chen, "Aromatherapy Benefits Autonomic Nervous System Regulation for Elementary School Faculty in Taiwan."

20. Jellinek, "Odours and Mental States," 115–20.

21. Marofi et al., "Evaluation of the Effect of Aromatherapy with *Rosa Damascena* Mill. on Postoperative Pain Intensity in Hospitalized Children in Selected Hospitals Affiliated to Isfahan University of Medical Sciences in 2013," 247–54.

22. Herz, "The Role of Odor-Evoked Memory in Psychological and Physiological Health," 22; Herz, "A Naturalistic Analysis of Autobiographical Memories Triggered by Olfactory Visual and Auditory Stimuli," 217–24.

23. Pitman, "Aromatherapy and Children with Learning Difficulties," 20–23.

CHAPTER 4.
COMPLEMENTARY WELLNESS TECHNIQUES

1. U.S. Department of Health and Human Services and U.S. Department of Agriculture, *2015–2020 Dietary Guidelines for Americans,* 8th edition, December 2015, https://health.gov/dietaryguidelines/2015 /resources/2015-2020_Dietary_Guidelines.pdf; Auestad and Fulgoni, "What Current Literature Tells Us about Sustainable Diets," 19–36; Rosi et al., "Environmental Impact of Omnivorous, Ovo-lacto-vegetarian, and Vegan Diet."

CONCLUSION

1. Gibran, *The Prophet,* 91.

Bibliography

Alexander, Michael. "How Theories of Motivation Apply to Olfactory Aromatherapy." *International Journal of Aromatherapy* 10, no. 3–4 (2001): 135–51.

Auestad, Nancy, and Victor L. Fulgoni III. "What Current Literature Tells Us about Sustainable Diets: Emerging Research Linking Dietary Patterns, Environmental Sustainability, and Economics." *Advances in Nutrition* 6, no. 1 (January 2015): 19–36. https://doi.org/10.3945/an.114.005694.

Ballard, Clive G., John T. O'Brien, Katharina Reichelt, and Elaine K. Perry. "Aromatherapy as a Safe and Effective Treatment for the Management of Agitation in Severe Dementia: The Results of a Double-Blind Placebo-Controlled Trial with Melissa." *Journal of Clinical Psychiatry* 63, no. 7 (2002): 553–58.

Beauregard, Mario. "Mind Does Really Matter: Evidence from Neuroimaging Studies of Emotional Self-Regulation, Psychotherapy, and Placebo Effect." *Progress in Neurobiology* 81, no. 4 (2007): 218–36.

Beshara, Mary C., and Diane Giddings. "Use of Plant Essential Oils in Treating Agitation in a Dementia Unit." *International Journal of Aromatherapy* 12, no. 4 (2002): 207–12.

Brand, Russel. *Revolution*. London: Random House, 2014.

Buchbauer, Gerhard, Leopold Jirovetz, Walter Jager, Christine Plank, and Hermann Dietrich. "Fragrance Compounds and Essential Oils with Sedative Effects upon Inhalation." *Journal of Pharmaceutical Science* 82, no. 6 (1993): 660–64.

Burch, Vidyamala. "The Mindful Way to Well Being: The Breathworks Approach." Breathworks for Living Well. 2010. www.breathworks-mind fulness.org.uk/PDF/Breathworks_mindfulness_article_Jan_2010.pdf (accessed May 20, 2018).

Busse, Daniela, Philipp Kudella, Nana-Marie Gruning, Gunter Gisselmann, Sonja Stander, Thomas Luger, Frank Jacobson, et al. "A Synthetic Sandalwood Odorant Induces Wound Healing Process in Human Keratinocytes via the Olfactory Receptor OR2AT4." *Journal of Investigative Dermatology* 134, no. 11 (2014): 2823–32.

Carmody, James. "Evolving Conceptions of Mindfulness in Clinical Settings." *Journal of Cognitive Psychotherapy* 23, no. 3 (2009): 270–80.

Chambers, Richard, Eleonora Gullone, and Nicholas B. Allen. "Mindful Emotion Regulation: An Integrative Review." *Clinical Psychology Review* 29, no. 6 (2009): 560–72.

Chang, Kang-Ming, and Chuh-Wei Chen. "Aromatherapy Benefits Autonomic Nervous System Regulation for Elementary School Faculty in Taiwan." *Evidenced-Based Alternative and Complementary Medicine* 2011, Article ID 946537 (2011). http://dx.doi.org/10.1155/2011/946537.

Clarkson, Petruska. *Gestalt Counselling in Action.* 2nd ed. London: Sage Publications, 1999.

Cordon, Shari L., Kirk W. Brown, and Pamela R. Gibson. "The Role of Mindfulness Based Stress Reduction on Perceived Stress: Preliminary Evidence for the Moderating Role of Attachment Style." *Journal of Cognitive Psychotherapy* 23, no. 3 (2009): 258–69.

Culpeper, Nicholas. *The English Physitian Enlarged: With Three Hundred, Sixty and Nine Medicines, Made of English Herbs That Were Not in Any Impression Untill This, Being an Astrologo-physical Discourse of the Vulgar Herbs of This Nation . . .* London: John Streater, 1666.

Damian, Peter, and Kate Damian. *Aromatherapy: Scent and Psyche; Using Essential Oils for Physical and Emotional Well-being.* Rochester, Vt.: Healing Arts Press, 1995.

Davenport, Liam. "Dietary Change Key to Improving Mental Health, Experts Say." Medscape. September 26, 2015. www.medscape.com /viewarticle/851553#vp_1.

Friedmann, Terry S. "Attention Deficit and Hyperactivity Disorder (ADHD)." *Essential Science Publishing,* 2001. http://files.meetup.com/1481956

/ADHD%20Research%20by%20Dr.%20Terry%20Friedmann.pdf (accessed May 21, 2018).

Fromm, Erich. *The Art of Listening.* Edited and with a foreword by Rainer Funk. New York: Continuum, 1994. Reprint, London: Constable, 1998. Page references are to the 1998 edition.

Gabriel, Lynne. *Speaking the Unspeakable.* New York: Routledge, 2005.

Gattefosse, Rene-Maurice. *Aromatherapy.* Translated and edited by Robert B. Tisserand. Saffron Walden, U.K.: CW Daniel Co., 1995.

Gibran, Kahlil. *The Prophet.* London: William Heinemann, 1980.

Godfrey, Heather. "Aromatherapy: Purely Simply, Effectively; Boundaries of Professional Practice." *International Journal of Clinical Aromatherapy* (2011).

———. "Counselling: A Journey in Experiential Learning." *Aromatherapy Times* 1, no. 65 (2005): 10–12.

———. "Counselling Skills: An Inseparable Aspect of Therapeutic Relationships." *Aromatherapy Times* 1, no. 55 (2002): 28–31.

———. "Essential Oils: Complementary Treatment for Attention Deficit Hyperactive Disorder." *International Journal of Clinical Aromatherapy* 6, no. 1 (2009): 14–22.

Goldin, Philippe, Wiveka Ramel, and James Gross. "Mindfulness Meditation Training and Self-Referential Processing in Social Anxiety Disorder: Behavioral and Neural Effects." *Journal of Cognitive Psychotherapy* 23, no. 3 (2009): 242–57.

Griffin, Christine A., Kimberly A. Kafadar, and Grace K. Pavlath. "MOR23 Promotes Muscle Regeneration and Regulates Cell Adhesion and Migration." *Developmental Cell* 17, no. 5 (2009): 649–61.

Gruner, O. Cameron, ed. and trans. *A Treatise on the Canon of Medicine of Avicenna.* New York: AMS Press, 1973.

Gunaratana, Bhante H. *Beyond Mindfulness: In Plain English.* Boston: Wisdom Publications, 2009.

Hanh, Thich Nhat. *The Miracle of Mindfulness.* London: Rider, 1991.

Haze, Shinichiro, Keiko Sakai, and Yoko Gozu. "Effects of Fragrance Inhalation on Sympathetic Activity in Normal Adults." *Japanese Journal of Pharmacology* 90, no. 3 (2002): 247–53.

Herz, Rachel "A Naturalistic Analysis of Autobiographical Memories Triggered by Olfactory Visual and Auditory Stimuli." *Chemical Senses* 29, no. 3 (2004): 217–24. https://doi.org/10.1093/chemse/bjh025.

———. "The Role of Odor-Evoked Memory in Psychological and Physiological Health." *Brain Sciences* 6, no. 3 (2016): 22. http://doi.org/10.3390 /brainsci6030022.

Holzel, Britta K., James Carmody, Mark Vangel, Christina Congleton, Sita M. Yerramsetti, Tim Gard, and Sara W. Lazar. "Mindfulness Practice Leads to Increases in Regional Brain Gray Matter Density." *Psychiatry Research: Neuroimaging* 191, no. 1 (2011): 36–43.

Ilmberger, Josef, Eva Heuberger, Claudia Mahrhofer, Heidrun Dessovic, Dietlinde Kowarik, and Gerhard Buchbauer. "The Influence of Essential Oils on Human Attention. 1: Alertness." *Chemical Senses* 26, no. 3 (2001): 239–45.

Jellinek, J. Stephan. "Odours and Mental States." *International Journal of Aromatherapy* 4, no. 3 (1998–1999): 115–20.

Jimbo, Daiki, Yuki Kimura, Miyako Taniguchi, Masashi Inoue, and Katsuya Urakami. "Effect of Aromatherapy on Patients with Alzheimer's Disease." *Psychogeriatrics* 9, no. 4 (2009): 173–79.

Kabat-Zinn, Jon. "At Home in Our Bodies." Interview by Joan Duncan Oliver. September 2002. www.bemindful.org/kabatzinnart.htm.

———. "Coming to Our Senses: A Conversation with Jon Kabat-Zinn." Interview. *Inquiring Mind,* Fall 2004. www.inquiringmind.com/Articles /JonKabat.html (accessed May 20, 2018).

Kovar, K. A., B. Gropper, D. Friess, and H. P. Ammon. "Blood Levels of 1,8-cineole and Locomotor Activity of Mice after Inhalation and Oral Administration of Rosemary Oil." *Planta Medica* 53, no. 4 (1987): 315–18.

Kutz, Ilan, Joan Borysenko, and Herbert Benson. "Meditation and Psychotherapy: A Rationale for the Integration of Dynamic Psychotherapy, the Relaxation Response, and Mindfulness Meditation." *American Journal of Psychiatry* 142, no. 1 (1985): 1–8.

Lawrence, Brian M. *Essential Oils 1988–1991.* Wheaton, Ill.: Allured Publishing, 1993.

Mace, Chris. *Mindfulness and Mental Health: Therapy, Theory and Science.* London: Routledge, 2008.

Mackenzie, Corey S., Patricia A. Poulin, and Rhonda Seidman-Carlson. "A Brief Mindfulness Based Stress Reduction Intervention for Nurses and Nurse Aides." *Applied Nursing Research* 19, no. 2 (2006): 105–9.

Marofi, Maryam, Motahareh Sirousfard, Mahin Moeini, and Alireza Ghanadi.

"Evaluation of the Effect of Aromatherapy with *Rosa Damascena* Mill. on Postoperative Pain Intensity in Hospitalized Children in Selected Hospitals Affiliated to Isfahan University of Medical Sciences in 2013: A Randomized Clinical Trial." *Iran Journal of Nursing and Midwifery Research* 20, no. 2 (2015): 247–54. www.ncbi.nlm.nih.gov/pmc/articles/PMC4387651.

Mearns, Dave, and Brian Thorne. *Person-Centred Counselling in Action.* London: Sage Publications, 1999.

Mehta, Phiroz D. *Holistic Consciousness: Reflections of the Destiny of Humanity.* Shaftsbury, U.K.: Element Books, 1989.

Moss, Mark, Jenny Cook, Keith A. Wesnes, and Paul E. Ducket. "Aromas of Rosemary and Lavender Essential Oils Differentially Affect Cognition and Mood in Healthy Adults." *International Journal of Neuroscience* 113, no. 1 (2003): 15–38.

Moss, Mark, and Lorraine Oliver. "Plasma 1,8-cineole Correlates with Cognitive Performance following Exposure to Rosemary Essential Oil Aroma." *Therapeutic Advances in Psychopharmacology* 2, no. 3 (2012): 103–13. www.ncbi.nlm.nih.gov/pmc/articles/PMC3736918.

Muhammad, Ali. "Medicinal Flora in Holy Quran." Academia. www.academia.edu/7872565/Medicinal_Plants_in_The_Quran (accessed May 20, 2018).

National Institute for Mental Health. "Transforming the Understanding and Treatment of Mental Illness: Mental Health Medications." Last revised October 2016. www.nimh.nih.gov/health/publications/mental-health-medications/index.shtml.

Ong, Jason, and David Sholtes. "A Mindfulness-Based Approach to the Treatment of Insomnia." *Journal of Clinic Psychology* 66, no. 11 (2010): 1175–84.

Pengelly, Andrew, James Snow, Simon Y. Mills, Andrew B. Scholey, Keith A. Wesnes, and Leah Reeves Butler. "Short-Term Study on the Effects of Rosemary on Cognitive Function in an Elderly Population." *Journal of Medicinal Food* 15, no. 1 (2012): 10–17.

Perry, Elaine. "Aromatherapy for the Treatment of Alzheimer's Disease." *Journal of Quality Research in Dementia* 3 (2014).

Pipe, Teri B., Jennifer J. Bortz, Amylou Dueck, Debra Pendergast, Vicki Buchda, and Jay Summers. "Nurse Leader Mindfulness Meditation Program for Stress Management." *Journal of Nursing Administration* 39, no. 3 (2009): 130–37.

Pitman, Vicky. "Aromatherapy and Children with Learning Difficulties." *Aromatherapy Today* 15 (2000): 20–23.

Pluznick, Jennifer L., Dong-Jing Zou, Xiaohong Zhang, Qingshang Yan, Diego J. Rodriguez-Gil, Christoph Eisner, Erika Wells, et al. "Functional Expression of the Olfactory Signaling System in the Kidney." *Proceedings of the National Academy of Science* 106, no. 6 (2008): 2059–64.

Rinpoche, Sakyon Mipham. "How to Do Mindfulness Meditation." Lion's Roar. July 28, 2017. www.lionsroar.com/how-to-do-mindfulness-meditation.

Rogers, Carl. *A Way of Being.* New York: Houghton Mifflin, 1980.

Rosi, Alice, Pedro Mena, Nicoletta Pellegrini, et al. "Environmental Impact of Omnivorous, Ovo-lacto-vegetarian, and Vegan Diet." *Scientific Reports* 7, no. 6105 (2017). doi:10.1038/s41598-017-06466-8.

Ryan, Sheila. *Vital Practice Stories from the Healing Arts: The Homeopathic and Supervisory Way.* Henderson, Nev.: Sea Change, 2004.

Schnaubelt, Kurt. *Advanced Aromatherapy: The Science of Essential Oil Therapy.* Rochester, Vt.: Healing Arts Press, 1995.

Shapiro, Shauna. L., John A. Astin, Scott R. Bishop, and Matthew Cordova. "Mindfulness-Based Stress Reduction for Health Care Professionals: Results from a Randomized Trial." *International Journal of Stress Management* 12, no. 2 (2005): 164–76.

Shapiro, Shauna L., Gary E. R. Schwartz, and Craig Santerre. "Meditation and Positive Psychology." In *Handbook of Positive Psychology,* edited by C. R. Snyder and Shane Lopez, 632–645. New York: Oxford University Press, 2002.

Sheppard-Hanger, Sylla. *The Aromatherapy Practitioner Reference Manual.* 2 vols. Tampa, Fla.: Atlantic Institute of Aromatherapy, 1998.

Snyder, C. R., and Shane Lopez. "Mindfulness, Flow, and Spirituality: In Search of Optimal Experiences." In *Positive Psychology,* 243–62. London: Sage Publications, 2007.

Sorensen, Janina. "The Hormonal Activity of Vitex agnus-castus and Its Importance in Therapy." Pre-published lecture paper (forwarded to author 2001).

Spehr, Marc, Gunter Gisselmann, Alexandra Poplawski, Jeffrey A. Riffell, Christian H. Wetzel, Richard K. Zimmer, and Hanns Hatt. "Identification of a Testicular Odorant Receptor Mediating Human Sperm Chemotaxis." *Science* 299, no. 5615 (2003): 2054–58.

Stone, Alex. "Smell Turns Up in Unexpected Places." *New York Times.* October 13, 2014. www.nytimes.com/2014/10/14/science/smell-turns-up -in-unexpected-places.html?_r=0.

Tisserand, Robert. *The Art of Aromatherapy.* Saffron Walden, U.K.: CW Daniel Co., 1997.

Tisserand, Robert, and Rodney Young. *Essential Oil Safety: A Guide for Health Professionals.* 2nd ed. London: Churchill Livingstone, 2014.

Valentine, Katie. "Americans Should Consider Eating Less Meat for Environmental Reasons, Scientists Say." ThinkProgress. February 20, 2015. https://thinkprogress.org/americans-should-consider-eating-less-meat-for -environmental-reasons-scientists-say-1e47c83af400.

Valnet, Jean. *The Practice of Aromatherapy.* Saffron Walden, U.K.: CW Daniel Co., 1996.

Wang, Danny J. J., Hengyi Rao, Marc Korczykowski, Nancy Wintering, John Pluta, Dharma S. Khalsa, and Andrew B. Newberg. "Cerebral Blood Flow Changes Associated with Different Meditation Practices and Perceived Depth of Meditation." *Psychiatry Research: Neuroimaging* 191 (2010): 60–67.

Werbach, Melvin R. "Nutritional Influence on Aggressive Behavior." *Journal of Orthomolecular Medicine* 7, no. 1 (1995): 45–51.

Williams, David G. *The Chemistry of Essential Oils: An Introduction for Aromatherapists, Beauticians, Retailers and Students.* Weymouth, England: Michelle Press, 2006.

———. *Lecture Notes on Essential Oils.* London: Eve Taylor, 2000.

Index

pyridoxine, 113

Rawat, Prem, 25, 26
relaxation techniques, 102
remedial massage, 109
research evidence
    on effects of essential oils, 65–71
    on mindfulness meditation, 22–25
resin burners, 93–95
riboflavin, 112
right brain processing, 51, 52
rites and rituals, 36
Rogers, Carl, 16
Rolf, Ida, 108
rolfing, 108
roller bottles, 83–84
room vaporizers, 64, 90–93
rose, 55, 56, 62, 70, 91
rosemary, 66, 67, 68

Sakyong Mipham Rinpoche, 20
secondary processing, 21
sedative effects, 66
selenium, 121
self-massage, 97–99
semantic mechanism, 69, 70
senses, miracle of, 13
Serenity Essential Oils, 9, 35–36
    characteristics of, 58–59
    limbic system and, 55–56, 60–64
    multidynamic qualities of, 64
    psycho-emotional action of, 60–63
Shapiro, Shauna L., 15, 19, 22
skin absorption, 41–43
skin reactions, 76, 77
slouching, 105
smell, sense of. *See* olfactory system

sodium, 116
solvent extraction, 31
spikenard, 63
steam diffusers, 90–91, 92
steam distillation, 30
steam inhalation, 88–90
sulfur, 117
sympathetic nervous system, 69

tea tree, 60
thalamus, 50, 56
thiamine, 112
Tisserand, Robert, vii
tissues for inhalation, 86–88
top notes, 56, 57–58
trace minerals, 118–22
trachea, 44, 45
Transcendental Meditation, ix

ultradian rhythm, 100–101
University of Salford, viii

vacuum distillation, 31
vaporizers, 64, 90–93
vegetarian diet, 110
venous capillaries, 47
vetivert, 63, 67
vitamins, 112–16

waking up, 19
wellness techniques. *See* complementary
    wellness techniques
wordlessness, 12–13

yoga, 29, 106

zinc, 118

About the Author

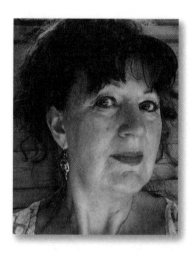

Heather studied at the University of Salford, where she was awarded a joint honors degree in counseling and complementary medicine, and master's certificates in integrated mindfulness and supervision of counseling and therapeutic relationships. She also gained a postgraduate teaching certificate from Bolton Institute. She worked at the College of Health and Social Care at the University of Salford for a number of years, fulfilling multiple roles. She served as a program lead and lecturer in integrated therapy, complementary therapy, aromatherapy, communication, and professional skills.

Heather has had a number of articles and research papers published in associated professional journals, including the *International Journal of Clinical Aromatherapy* (IJCA). A fellow of the International Federation of Aromatherapists (IFA), she was chair of education during 2013 and supports the IFA's educational program in an advisory capacity and as an examiner. She is also a member of the Federation of Holistic Therapists (FHT). Through her private practice, Heather continues to provide professional training, essential oil therapy treatments, professional supervision for therapists, professional development, and introductory workshops. Visit her website at

www.aromantique.co.uk.

BOOKS OF RELATED INTEREST

The Healing Intelligence of Essential Oils
The Science of Advanced Aromatherapy
by Kurt Schnaubelt, Ph.D.

Advanced Aromatherapy
The Science of Essential Oil Therapy
by Kurt Schnaubelt, Ph.D.

Essential Oils in Spiritual Practice
Working with the Chakras, Divine Archetypes,
and the Five Great Elements
by Candice Covington
Foreword by Sheila Patel, M.D.

Aromatherapy for Healing the Spirit
Restoring Emotional and Mental Balance with Essential Oils
by Gabriel Mojay

The Art of Aromatherapy
The Healing and Beautifying Properties of
the Essential Oils of Flowers and Herbs
by Robert B. Tisserand

Holistic Reflexology
Essential Oils and Crystal Massage in Reflex Zone Therapy
by Ewald Kliegel

Total Life Cleanse
A 28-Day Program to Detoxify and Nourish the Body, Mind, and Soul
by Jonathan Glass, M.Ac., C.A.T.

Natural Antibiotics and Antivirals
18 Infection-Fighting Herbs and Essential Oils
by Christopher Vasey, N.D.

INNER TRADITIONS • BEAR & COMPANY
P.O. Box 388
Rochester, VT 05767
1-800-246-8648
www.InnerTraditions.com

Or contact your local bookseller

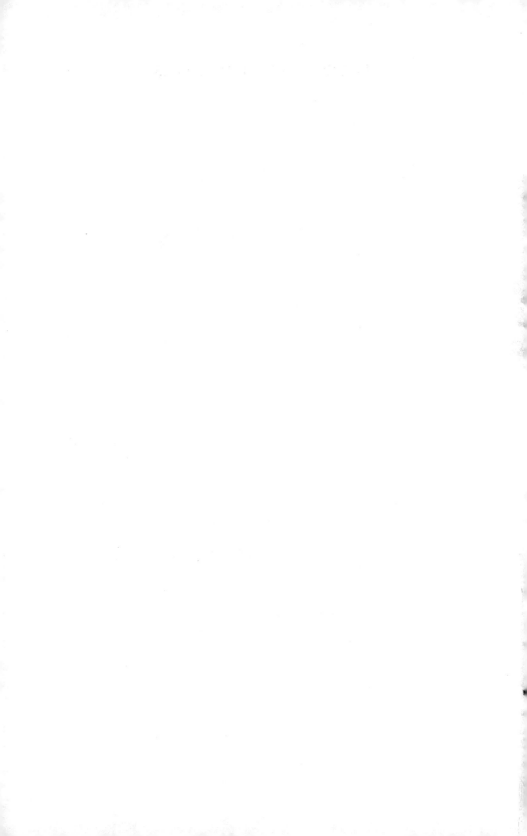